Penny and Andrew Stanway are London-trained doctors who were married in 1969. They have three children and live in Surrey.

Penny Stanway has spent some time in general practice, research and as Senior Medical Officer to a large Area Health Authority. Her main interest now lies in helping women to breastfeed their babies successfully and she is on the Professorial Advisory Board of La Leche League International. She writes on baby and child care for various magazines and journals and has written three books with her husband.

Andrew Stanway, MB, MRCP, was a medical registrar at a London teaching hospital until 10 years ago. He now lectures, broadcasts, writes and makes films on medical topics, both for the medical profession and for the general public. He has written ten books including titles on nutrition and child care. *Breast is Best*, written jointly with his wife, has become an international best seller.

Also by Drs Penny and Andrew Stanway

Breast is Best
The Pears Encyclopaedia of Child Health

By Dr Andrew Stanway

Taking the Rough with the Smooth
The Boots book of First Aid
Alternative Medicine - a guide to Natural Therapies
A Dictionary of Operations
Why Us? A common-sense guide for the childless
Overcoming Depression

Drs Penny and Andrew Stanway

THE BREAST

Illustrated by Giovanni Casselli

A MAYFLOWER BOOK

GRANADA
London Toronto Sydney New York

Published by Granada Publishing Limited 1982

ISBN 0 583 13464 5

A Granada Paperback Original
Copyright © Drs Penny and Andrew Stanway 1982

Granada Publishing Limited
Frogmore, St Albans, Herts AL2 2NF
and
36 Golden Square, London W1R 4AH
366 United Nations Plaza, New York, NY 10017, USA
117 York Street, Sydney, NSW 2000, Australia
100 Skyway Avenue, Rexdale, Ontario, M9W 3A6, Canada
61 Beach Road, Auckland, New Zealand

Printed and bound in Great Britain
by Richard Clay Ltd,
Bungay, Suffolk
Set in Plantin

Granada ®
Granada Publishing ®

Contents

Acknowledgements

We should like to thank:
The National Childbirth Trust
La Leche League
The Mastectomy Association
The Librarian and Staff of the Royal Society of Medicine
Dr Philip Cauthery
Dr David Clayden
Many of the senior staff of Berlei UK Ltd
Mr Cyril Young FRCS, MRCOG
Mr Peter Howie FRCOG
Mr Brian Hogbin FRCS
and the many women who have talked and written to us so freely.

Our special thanks to Dr Henry Patrick Leis Jr, Clinical Professor of
Surgery and Chief of the Breast Service, New York Medical College,
Valhalla, New York, USA, who checked through the final draft of the
book and wrote the Foreword.

Foreword

THE BREAST, by Drs Andrew and Penny Stanway, deals with all important aspects of the breast, presenting in a precise and easy-to-read fashion its psychological and physical importance. The magnificent section on breastfeeding is a must for every woman to read; the common, benign problems that cause concern among many women are well presented and should help to remove many of the misunderstandings that pertain to these lesions; the chapter on breast self-examination is excellent; and there is a good discussion of the various diagnostic aids that can be utilized in evaluating breast problems.

Breast cancer is presented in a non-alarming fashion, the authors emphasizing the fine results that can be obtained with appropriate surgery and selective adjuvant therapy. The importance of early diagnosis is forcibly brought home – early diagnosis results not only in better cure rates, but also in less extensive surgery, less adjuvant therapy and better cosmetic and functional results. In the United States, the most commonly used operation today is a conservative modified radical mastectomy, rather than simple mastectomy or more radical procedures. This operation removes the entire breast and axillary nodes but preserves the pectoral muscles, and was the procedure recommended by the National Institute of Health Consensus Conference in 1979 for patients with Stage I and selected Stage 2 breast cancers.

The section on bras is outstanding and the book even has a section on the male breast which brings into clear focus the important aspects of both benign and malignant lesions as they affect the male.

This book represents a monumental collection of knowledge gleaned from thousands of women, and it is one that should be in the library of everybody's home.

HENRY PATRICK LEIS, Jr., MD.
Clinical Professor of Surgery and Chief of the
Breast Service; Co-director, Institute of Breast

Diseases, New York Medical College, Valhalla,
N.Y. Chief of Breast Surgery, Cabrini Medical
Centre, New York City.

CHAPTER 1

Breasts in society

We decided to write *The Breast* soon after the publication of our bestselling book on breastfeeding, *Breast is Best*. It is impossible to come into contact with thousands of women in the context of breast-feeding-counselling and not to become aware of the extraordinary feelings women have about their breasts. Many of the current attitudes towards and reasons for the failure of breastfeeding arise because so many of us, men and women, have such peculiar notions about breasts. There can scarcely be an organ of the body of either sex that arouses such powerful emotions − except perhaps the penis but this is by and large a hidden piece of a man's anatomy and is not his most obvious sexual symbol, except when undressed.

In today's society, with women's hair generally shorter, with women wearing trousers and competing with men in all spheres of life, a woman's breasts are often just about the only obvious sexual signal that immediately distinguishes her from her male partner. Quite understandably, a society which is still substantially male-dominated has put an over-emphasis on women's breasts for this very reason.

The biological perspective

As a species, humans develop breasts (and quite large ones for their size compared with other animals) very early. Most mammals only develop their mammary glands in time to feed their young, but human beings, whose breasts are well developed several years before childbearing begins, even in hunter-gatherers and other traditional rural peoples, clearly have them for other purposes too. The chief among these is almost certainly as a source of sexual arousal in a species of mammal that (along with the other higher primates) is unusual in wanting to and being able to copulate at any time. The vast majority of the animal kingdom's sexual activities revolve around times during which the female can be fertilized and only then if she is interested in (or even in some cases capable of) intercourse. Humans, on the other hand, are interested in sexual intercourse from soon after puberty until death and, apart from periods of physical and mental illness, are capable of having intercourse several times in one day let alone a handful of times a year as with many animal species.

All this means that intercourse has come to have a different significance to humans — it is a source of pleasure which is not necessarily related to procreation.

Human beings have probably been on the face of the earth for about five million years, and until five thousand years ago lived as hunter-gatherers, eating like apes a vegetarian diet. It seems from such evidence as is available from historical remains and from the study of the few hunter-gatherer tribes that persist in the world today that the whole reproductive life of such people is very different from our own. Perhaps the best-studied hunter-gatherers of the present day are the !Kung of Botswana and Namibia who live as our ancestors are thought to have lived for millions of years. Their women menstruate late by Western standards (at about seventeen to eighteen) and their menopause is earlier — at about thirty-eight. Their total female reproductive span is therefore only about twenty years long, whereas ours is about thirty-six years (between the ages of thirteen and forty-nine). Also, because they breastfeed their young on an unrestricted basis they do not ovulate for much of their reproductive lives and so do not menstruate, often for years on end. Women who live like this (as indeed all of humanity did until about five thousand years ago when they started living in settlements based on agricultural food supplies) become fertile, menstruate a few times, have their first child whom they breastfeed for several years and then, when their ovulation returns as breastfeeding falls off, become pregnant again and so repeat the cycle. To such women, menstruation is not a monthly event but an uncommon one which occurs as a result of their relatively few ovulatory cycles. They have perhaps six or seven children, some of whom die at birth or during the first year, and so end up with a family of three or four children.

So the overall pattern was that hunter-gatherer women were either pregnant or breastfeeding for almost the whole of their reproductive lives. This in turn meant that instead of experiencing the 400-450 menstrual cycles of the modern Western woman they only had 20-30 in a whole lifetime.

This then was the picture until a mere 5,000 years ago — a blink of an eye in terms of evolution. Biologically we are still more akin to these hunter-gatherers than to anyone else, yet over the past two hundred years of industrial society we have dramatically changed our way of life to one in which women start menstruating earlier, and have regular monthly menstrual cycles with accompanying surges of hormones on hundreds of occasions until the menopause intervenes at about the age of fifty. Changes were, of course, occurring over many thousands of years but it seems that our very recent change in lifestyle has accelerated things considerably.

Just what all this does to modern woman we don't yet know but we can be sure that her body wasn't made to cope with such abnormal patterns. Our females' reproductive systems have evolved to behave in one way yet today's life-style forces them to behave in quite another.

'But,' we can hear you say, 'all these hunter-gatherers must have had a child every three or four years, spaced only by their breast-feeding contraception. I don't want a child every three years, so what relevance has all this for me?' Certainly this is a valid point. The human reproductive system can compensate for very considerable wastage. Human females have one of the highest levels of fetal wastage (miscarriage) of any animal and also lose many babies at and soon after birth especially without medical intervention. The hunter-gatherer type of reproductive pattern in the past and that of many Third World peoples today compensates for this considerable wastage. Today in the West, though, when the vast majority of children live, even if women were pregnant or breastfeeding for much of the time as hunter-gatherer women were, the result would be families larger than society would consider acceptable.

What, though, has all this to do with a book on the breast? Quite simply the breast is an integral part of a woman's reproductive system. Her breasts are linked into the same hormonal systems that operate during orgasm, childbirth, breastfeeding and her menstrual cycles — in other words, during her whole reproductive life. We shall see later that all these are closely interlinked in a woman's whole biological functioning.

There is very little doubt that breast cancer (now the commonest cancer killer in women) has become more common over the last two hundred years and that benign (non-cancerous) conditions of the breast are enormously common. It has been estimated that one in fourteen women in the West today will get breast cancer and that one in *four* will suffer from some sort of breast condition or disease.

Why should this be? Why should women's breasts be so prone to disease? The answer probably lies in the extraordinary way that we treat them – a way which is so recent in evolutionary terms that our bodies haven't had a chance to adapt to it. Breastfeeding is still the single most important method of contraception around the world yet few women in the so-called 'enlightened' West realize it. By breastfeeding so little or even not at all we rob the breasts of one of their main functions and the high incidence of breast disorders may be the price we are paying. And it's not only the breast that's suffering. Endometrial cancer (cancer of the lining of the uterus) is clearly linked to the incidence of breast cancer, so perhaps the 450 menstrual cycles today's modern Western woman experiences in her lifetime are playing havoc with her uterus too. After all, each month, if she is ovulating, a woman's body gets ready for a pregnancy. Her breasts, uterus and ovaries undergo profound physiological and anatomical changes (as we shall see on page 49. Many of these changes involve the growth of new cells and the stimulation of cellular ribonucleic acid (RNA). It's but a short step in cellular terms from the repeated normal overgrowth of cells to their abnormal overgrowth in the form of a cancer. The whole system is keyed up ready for the fertilization of the egg each month. In our modern world, however, eggs are fertilized only once or twice in about 450 cycles (compared with seven or eight times in thirty cycles in hunter-gatherer women): all the other cycles are 'wasted' in biological terms. This would be no great tragedy if it weren't for the fact that these profound bodily changes are repeatedly being frustrated year after year and that clearly they weren't meant to be. This may be why modern woman has such an enormous amount of reproductive organ illness. Cancer of the breast and endometrium are alarmingly common and one in five women in the UK ends up having her uterus removed – can this be normal or desirable? Few babies are breast-fed for nearly long enough, robbing them of the provable advantages of breastfeeding that go way beyond simple nutrition – can this be right?

So without being unnecessarily doom-laden we are faced with some pretty horrifying facts, and our modern life seems to be geared to perpetuating the horrors rather than to alleviating them.

What can be done then to try to redress the balance, at least a little?

There's very little we can do in 1981 to make girls start menstruating later. It has been found that the age at first menstruation is linked to the nutritional status of a community so perhaps by stopping *over-nourishing* our children we could delay puberty, if only for a few years eventually.

Once a girl starts menstruating she should ideally start having children within a very few years. As we shall see, one of the greatest proven preventives against breast cancer is having a first baby young (under twenty). The female reproductive system wasn't designed to function for a decade or more before its first baby and if we continue to insist that it does, we'll continue to have problems. This at first sight entails a complete change in society which is unlikely to come about rapidly, if at all. What is likely is that the pharmaceutical companies will develop synthetically-produced hormones that mimic those produced by the pituitary gland of the woman who is constantly pregnant or breastfeeding. Work is under way to isolate and prepare such substances. When such a compound exists a girl could keep her hormone profile in such a state that she would not ovulate. Many women wonder why, since the Pill prevents ovulation, it could not be used to achieve just this, especially in the light of the fact that women on the Pill seem to have far fewer benign (non-cancerous) breast conditions than do other women. The answer is that the Pill is such a therapeutic blunderbuss and has so many undesirable metabolic effects that it could not be used for twenty years or more in any one woman. On the contrary, all recent research and publicity have tended to make women come off the Pill and not to go on it for long periods! No, a specially tailor-made hormone-type preparation would have to be used which would prevent ovulation yet have no undesirable actions in a woman's body. Once she was rendered an-ovulatory in this way she would then behave biologically like the !Kung and her hunter-gatherer ancestors and would almost certainly have fewer breast and other reproductive ailments and diseases. Anovulation isn't the whole answer though because it is possible that the hormonal changes of pregnancy and breastfeeding may be protective too.

Of course, the ideal answer would be for women to go back to a more natural pattern of reproduction but this is unlikely to occur in the foreseeable future unless society changes dramatically for some reason. Few societies in the world today can afford the increase in population that would go with a return to such a reproductive lifestyle.

Once a woman starts having babies her whole reproductive system *can* be influenced, if only for a few years, by breastfeeding on an *unrestricted* basis, as often as the baby wants the breast. Nutritionally; it is usually unnecessary to breastfeed much beyond eight months or so in the Western world but from the *woman's* point of view there is every reason for carrying on with very frequent feeds, even if the child is getting much of its nourishment from adult-type foods. With very frequent nipple stimulation the mother's hormones remain at levels which prevent ovulation. This not only acts as a natural contraceptive but also prevents the monthly changes which, as we have seen, may be harmful when repeated year after year.

In this way the woman could enjoy a year or more of post-baby anovulation and this, together with nine months of pregnancy, gives her two years or so per baby of more biologically normal reproductive behaviour. Even two children per woman then gives four years of protection and it's possible that the benefits in biological terms increase with the more children she has, provided they are all breast-fed for a long time.

The current situation with women's reproductive ills is hardly ideal and with the probable decreasing need for people to work over the next few decades perhaps we shall see a return to more biological mothering, earlier childbearing and, who knows, even a return to a more stable family life as a result. We live in a world geared to women behaving totally abnormally in biological terms and we are probably paying the price in many ways — not the least in breast disease.

A historical view

The breast has always enchanted humanity because of its importance in the propagation and preservation of the species, and it has inspired artists and sculptors since Palaeolithic times.

The ancient Hebrew compilers of the Talmud believed that in girls of wealthier families the right breast developed earlier than the left, since they wore their shawls on the right side and this kept the right half of the chest warmer, so favouring the growth of the right breast. But among girls born to poorer people the left breast developed sooner because they lifted water pitchers with their left hands and carried their little brothers and sisters on their left arms.

Throughout history people have attempted to shape and mould young girls' breasts and Ploss and Bartels, the distinguished anthropologists, reported that among South African rural peoples, for example, the breasts were carefully treated and developed. When their daughters were as young as eight years old mothers began to rub their breasts with ointment made from grease and certain roots, then, 'they grasped the areola and sensitive portions around the nipple and rubbed and kneaded them as though they wanted to tear off the whole gland'. At a later stage the nipple was elongated and tied around with strips of fibre. In parts of New Guinea the breasts of growing girls have been subjected to extraordinary treatments and superstitious practices, including the inducing of swelling with nettles and ants.

Several African tribes have customs which involve constricting the breasts by means of a band across the top tied so tightly that the breasts are held down. This must affect their development. No one knows why this is done but in a very few years full, firm breasts subjected to such treatment become flaccid and pendulous. In many areas of the world breast flattening and elongation are practised as a matter of course.

In Europe in the sixteenth and seventeenth centuries Spanish women practised a strange custom on their young girls. At puberty their breasts were covered with lead plates which resulted in a chest concavity rather than a prominence. Extreme thinness was considered beautiful at the time, leading Countess d'Aulnoy to remark with pride that her breasts were 'as flat and even as a sheet of paper'. Many other European countries, until quite recent times, forced their young girls into constricting garments to flatten the breasts. This compression meant that very little glandular tissue formed and that the women could not feed their babies. Many babies undoubtedly died as a result of this fashion unless they were wet-nursed.

Over the centuries and around the world the breast has been variously tattooed, adorned and mutilated. Certain African tribes still scar the breasts as a form of decoration though this used to be very much more popular than it is today. In various places at various times the nipples have been mutilated so as to make them unsuitable for suckling and all kinds of strange practices have been carried out in small country towns in Europe in recent centuries. Even today nipple piercing to take rings and other jewellery is not at all uncommon in Western cultures.

Certain religious groups in the past sought to obliterate the breasts of young novices and nuns so that they would be 'like the angels', neither male nor female. The Amazon women are, of course, legendary in this way too. They had their right breast removed in childhood so that they could draw a bow and hunt effectively. Their breasts were removed by making a brass disc red hot and pressing it on the right breast until the flesh and muscles were so damaged that they would never develop.

As late as the nineteenth century mutilations were practised by the Skoptsi, an obscure Christian sect chiefly of Russian origin. These people went in for genital mutilation and also cut off the nipples of girls aged nine or ten. Their form of divine service seems to have included a ritual supper at which a small portion of a girl's mutilated breast was devoured instead of the Host.

Perhaps the most lingering legend arising out of the attempts in all parts of the Christian world to obliterate these conspicuous signs of womanly beauty so as to direct men's minds from things of this earth was that of the Sicilian virgin Agatha, who lived in Catania in the first half of the third century. Consul Quintianus wooed her to be his wife but she refused him. He then imprisoned her in a brothel where she was tortured by having her breasts mutilated. Her feast day is celebrated on 5 February and wax images of her breasts are carried in her honour in Sicily to this day.

Human milk has had magical properties attributed to it and has been recommended for treating conditions as different as deafness and snakebites. Conversely there have been widespread beliefs that lactation was governed by supernatural forces, and amulets and chains have been used all over the world by nursing women to increase their milk supply and by farmers to increase milk yields in their animals. There was a legend popular in Imperial Rome that the Grecian Pero daily visited her aged father Micon in prison where she breast-fed him and saved him from death by starvation. This legend, with the theme 'Caritas Romana' (Roman charity), has been popularized in pottery, mural paintings and terracotta statuettes in Pompeii. The city prison in Ghent has a relief dating from 1741 depicting the girl breastfeeding her father. It was replaced by a copy (because the old one was so badly weathered) as recently as the 1960s.

Today the breast has a more overt sexual significance that is little tinged with religious guilt. Most Western women, while only too happy to admit that their breasts are capable of feeding infants, choose to ignore this function and so relegate them to a solely sexual one. We don't show our genitals. Except when wearing very tight jeans most women don't use their buttocks as sexual symbols. The fall from grace of lipstick has meant that the mouth is no longer the sexual focal point it was. As a result breasts, especially in the USA, reign supreme as sex symbols in men's eyes. Without doubt the breast has overtaken all other parts of the human anatomy in this respect, leading to an unnatural sexual emphasis on breasts in our society. Quite understandably many modern women find this difficult to accept — and with good reason.

About our research

Over the years we've been involved in talking to women about their breasts we've quite naturally become very aware of most of the things that concern women about them. But even so, we found there were areas that are rarely discussed and on which the medical literature is scanty or non-existent. In late 1980 we therefore created a question- naire which we gave to three hundred women of all social classes to try to remedy some of these defects. We asked the women not only to fill in the questionnaire (which was totally anonymous) but also to write in freehand anything else they felt strongly about their breasts. Many of the respondents took the opportunity to write extra comments, and some expressed gratitude that we were bothering to find out what women actually felt.

Before we look in detail at the findings of our research let's just outline the profile of those who responded. The sample was somewhat biased in that over half of the women were single (51 per cent) and that 85 per cent were under forty. The relative youth of our sample arose from the way we recruited our subjects. We placed advertisements in women's magazines and gave questionnaires to women of our ac- quaintance (personal and professional). Clearly this tended to recruit a certain sort of woman but quite frankly there is no way of obtaining a 'balanced' sample for such a survey because we could never have compelled reluctant women to take part. Overall, there was a greater resistance among the over-forties to accept and complete the questionnaire but even in the under-forties there was still more resistance than we'd expected. A few husbands refused to allow their wives to answer the questionnaire at all – which said a lot about the whole subject and serves to remind anyone interested in such sensitive subjects that the level of sexual repression, even among the young, is still high. Some women were 'disgusted' by the whole idea, others sought confirmation from the periodical in which the ad appeared that we were bona fide doctors and so on. One major national daily newspaper even refused to carry our advertisement asking women to send off for a questionnaire! Overall, there was hostility from more people than we had imagined would be the case but this only confirmed our existing impressions – that many women are insecure about their breasts and are ill at ease with them. We shall look in more detail at what some of our respondents said about their breasts in a moment but first let's examine the questionnaire's findings.

In the first section entitled *Your Childhood and Adolescence* we tried to ascertain what women felt about the background that had produced their current attitudes to their breasts. Nearly three-quarters of our sample were breast-fed as babies – a surprisingly high percentage considering that most were born since World War II, a period not known for its high breastfeeding levels in society.

Forty per cent claimed that they had never been told anything about breasts at all as girls, but of those who had been informed on the subject, by far the most had been told by their mothers. *None* had discussed the subject with their fathers. The second commonest source of information was their school.

Three-quarters of the women claimed that as children they saw breasts as having a solely nutritional role. This is interesting because the vast majority of mature women certainly do not perceive this to be the case. Could it be that in the absence of any other perceived function a child sees nutrition as the only possible use for the breast? Whatever the explanation, as girls grow up their views on the major function of their breasts clearly change.

Women in our survey claimed that their breasts first developed at ages as different as eight and thirty-one, with the vast majority being between ten and fourteen, as would be expected. Just under a half (49 per cent) first developed breasts when they were eleven or twelve. The overwhelming feeling (bearing in mind that we were asking our women to cast their minds back and that they might not have remembered accurately) as their breasts developed was one of pleasure. Fifty-six per cent said they were 'pleased' but a third were 'shy' and 24 per cent 'embarrassed'. One in ten said they were 'worried' or 'unhappy' but we couldn't go any further into these negative feelings in a questionnaire such as this.

As young girls develop they touch their breasts out of curiosity and admiration and eventually as a part of sexual arousal and discovery. Well over 80 per cent claimed to have touched or looked at their breasts as they were developing and 81 per cent had compared their breasts with those of other women and girls.

It seems from our study that although most girls' breasts developed at about eleven or twelve they went a year or so before buying their first bra. More girls bought their first bra at the age of twelve than at any other age (27 per cent) but 24 per cent did so at thirteen and 21 per cent at fourteen. Two women bought their first bra at twenty-eight and one at over thirty.

It is well known in psychosexual circles that even quite young girls are very aware that their breasts are sexual symbols. To our surprise 20 per cent claimed to have tried to alter their breasts as they were growing. The vast majority of these had tried exercises but some had tried creams, massage, binding and other methods. Predictably (by us, but alas not by the girls at the time), 93 per cent said that what they had tried had done no good at all. While 20 per cent were trying to increase their bust size, 25 per cent were trying to hide their breasts. They did this by rounding their shoulders and by wearing certain clothes that hid their developing bust. Only a tiny number went so far as to bind their breasts.

About a quarter of the girls thought that their breast development had influenced their relationships with the girls around them and approximately half thought the influence had been for the better and half for the worse. When it came to boys things were, not surprisingly, different. Forty-two per cent felt that their developing breasts influenced the way they related to boys and twice as many found this produced an improvement in relationships rather than a deterioration. What is perhaps more interesting is that 50 per cent thought that their developing breasts hadn't had any effect on their relationship with boys.

A girl's first sexual experiences with her breasts are almost all homosexual, as we shall see in Chapter 4, but by the age of thirteen, one in five of our sample had already had their breasts touched over

their clothes by a boy. Over 40 per cent had experienced sexual
breast contact over their clothes by the age of fourteen, and by the age
of seventeen, 88 per cent of the girls had experienced breast contact in
sexual activities with boys. When it came to sex-play under clothes the
picture shows that half as many girls aged thirteen allowed boys to
play with their breasts under their clothes than over them, yet by the
age of sixteen these numbers had evened out. Remarkably, by today's
standards, just over one-third of the girls had experienced no
under-clothes sex play up to the age of seventeen. This figure would
probably be different if it were asked of seventeen-year-olds today.

In section two – *Your breasts today* – we tried to find out how
women felt about their breasts at the time of the questionnaire. It is so
widely held by the medical and corsetry worlds that women are
generally dissatisfied with their breasts that we wanted to see if this
were true. One quarter (23 per cent) said they were 'a bit dissatisfied'
and a third 'fairly satisfied', 15 per cent 'neither satisfied not
dissatisfied'; and only 19 per cent said they were 'highly satisfied'. So,
overall, there was definitely a tendency for our women to be dissatisfied with their breasts. We asked whether they'd like their breasts
to be different from how they are and 54 per cent said they would.
When asked how they thought most (other) women viewed their
breasts only 1.5 per cent said they thought other women were 'highly
satisfied' and only 20 per cent 'fairly satisfied' with them. Forty-three
per cent thought other women were 'a bit dissatisfied' with their breasts.

We wanted to know what our respondents thought their partners
felt about their breasts. Fascinatingly, although such a small proportion of our women were satisfied with their breasts, a very substantial proportion (48 per cent) thought that their partners were
'hightly satisfied' with them and another 23 per cent thought they were
'fairly satisfied'. We wonder what their partners themselves thought!
So although many of our women were dissatisfied with their own
breasts they obviously felt that their partners were more easily
pleased. Could this be wishful thinking or are women more critical of
their own breasts than they think men are? Only 15 per cent thought
their partners would want to alter their breasts if they could. Again, it
would have been interesting to have had the partners' views on this.

The overwhelming majority of women had never tried anything to
improve their breasts. Ninety per cent claimed never to have tried
anything in adult life that would improve their bust, but of the 10 per

cent who had, exercises were by far the most popular with plastic surgery, water splashes, creams and other methods coming way down the list. Of those who had tried anything, fewer than half claimed to have noticed any improvement.

Because modern society is influenced by the media, including the popular press and girlie magazines, in its view of what breasts should notionally look like we tried to find out what women saw as being the 'ideal' breast (to which most clearly thought they did not aspire, according to their previous answers!). We gave a choice of eight adjectives that are generally used when describing the breast. 'Firm' was the attribute overwhelmingly chosen (78 per cent) as most important, with 'needs no bra' (60 per cent) coming next. From a computer analysis of the answers we can conclude that in those women who had a concept of an 'ideal' shaped breast (and some found the whole idea quite silly and refused even to answer the question) this description was (in descending order of importance) firm, needs no bra, pointed nipples, and small. This then is the stereotype that our women felt they were not living up to when so many of them said they weren't pleased with their breasts.

When asked how their partners' concept of the 'ideal' breast fitted in with this it was found that twice as many men wanted 'large' breasts as their ideal compared with their women and that only about half as many as the women put stress on being able to go without a bra. 'Firm' was the first choice of the partners, with 'pointed nipple' and 'needs no bra' following close behind. Overall, most men seemed to be more easily pleased by a wider range of breast descriptions than did their owners.

Finally in this section we asked our respondents whether they thought that women in general worried too much about their breasts. In other words, was the book we were writing likely to hit on an area of real concern to women? Sixty-five per cent said that they thought women worried too much about their breasts.

Because the breast is such a potent sex symbol in human life and because this fact is often ignored or negated, we felt it important to find out first-hand in a totally anonymous way what women felt about the subject. Far too many sex experts have given their subjective interpretations of the subject but there is no substitute for going 'straight to the horse's mouth' for such information.

Section three of our survey was called *Breasts and sex*.

As so many women are supposed to be dissatisfied with their breasts (as our results confirmed) we asked if men liked their breasts. Nearly 60 per cent said that men generally did like their breasts and the other 40 per cent said they didn't know. Women were equally divided into those who cared whether men liked their breasts and those that did not care.

Our sample of women were also asked what men most often did to their breasts during lovemaking. Seventy per cent (the highest number) said 'kiss' and 68 per cent 'suck' with about half of the women saying that their men stroked or squeezed their breasts. These proportions presumably reflect what their partners most wanted to do, so we then asked what the women themselves most liked having done. Kissing came top of the list again but was not as popular as the men thought; stroking was enjoyed by over half of the women; but twice as many men squeezed their partners' breasts as wanted it done. Analysis showed that men like to do the following to their partner's breasts during lovemaking (in descending desirability order): kiss, suck, touch, stroke, squeeze, hold. Women, however, put the emphasis slightly differently: kiss, suck, stroke, touch, hold, squeeze.

Since it is well known that many women's breast-play preferences arise as a direct result of their masturbation practices we tried to find if this was in fact the case. In our sample 87 per cent answered the masturbation question and of those who did 47 per cent said that their breasts were involved as part of their masturbation pattern. Two-thirds of those whose breasts were important as a part of masturbation played with their nipples and 60 per cent stroked their breasts. Over a third squeezed their breast(s) and one in twenty sucked their nipples. It's interesting that half as many women again enjoyed squeezing their own breasts during masturbation as enjoyed having them squeezed during lovemaking. Perhaps there is a lesson here for men to learn how to squeeze their women's breasts in a way they enjoy.

It is well known that the female body is a sexual 'turn on' to both men and women but as far as we know no one has ever specifically sought women's opinions about the sexiness of other women's breasts. Thirty-five per cent of our respondents said that women's breasts made them sexually excited and 36 per cent said that they were 'turned on' by the pictures of women in the so-called 'men's magazines'. On the other side of the coin 45 per cent of the sample said that they thought such material was harmful, misleading or disgusting. About one in seven resented their partners looking at such pictures.

Although women's breasts are obviously erotic centres for both sexes a lot of speculation has gone on as to just how orgasmic an organ the breast is for most women. More than 17 per cent of women in our survey claimed that they could experience an orgasm with breast stimulation alone. This seems rather high compared with the experience of other researchers but may reflect the younger and more sexually at ease nature of the women in our sample.

Bras, the subject of our fourth section, are a very important item in almost every woman's wardrobe and women spend millions of pounds a year on them. Exactly three-quarters of our sample said that they usually wore a bra but an equal percentage also said either that they didn't much like wearing one or that they didn't mind one way or the other. Sixty-four per cent said that they sometimes went without a bra and 17 per cent always went without one. Nineteen per cent always wore a bra. When asked why they wore a bra, 'comfort' and 'support' came out equal tops, with 'appearance' a close third, but nearly half (49 per cent) found it difficult to get a bra they felt good in. The main complaints women had were (in this order) that it was difficult to find one they liked; difficult to get the bra they liked in their size; and 14 per cent thought it was difficult to get in-store help. Only just over a quarter found it easy to get a bra. Contrary to what many men think about women left to themselves not bothering to 'pretty themselves up', 60 per cent of women said they would wear a bra even if they lived entirely among women. This confirms previous findings of several studies that women wear bras to please themselves and for their own comfort. Most women felt that those who could go without a bra were 'lucky' yet when asked whether men liked it when they went bra-less 60 per cent said they didn't know and only 35 per cent said that men did.

Most women have never been fitted for a bra. Could this be a reason why so many women can't buy a bra they feel happy in? Only a third of our sample had ever been fitted for a bra. When it came to bra sizes 42 per cent were 34; 32 per cent 36; 7 per cent 38 and 2 per cent 40.

Section five was about *Health*. Eighty per cent of our sample had been on the Pill at some stage and over half had found that taking it had made no difference to the size of their breasts. However, 37 per cent said that their breasts had got bigger. 'Tenderness when touched' was the commonest side effect of the Pill on the breasts but there was no change in the women's sexual enjoyment from their breasts while taking it.

Almost 70 per cent of all the women said that their breasts changed with their monthly cycle, with 'more tender' being the main complaint. A quarter said that their breasts were painful even when they weren't touched and 40 per cent said they were bigger at some stage. Most changes took place a few days before a period and led many of the women to say that they didn't want their breasts touched at this time. Men, please note!

One in five of our women had had a breast lump and three-quarters of them discovered the lump themselves. Most went to a doctor within a few days though one in six waited a month or more. This is far sooner than average but again the youth of our sample could explain this. Eighty-five per cent claimed to feel their breasts for lumps but 79 per cent of these only did so 'from time to time'. Only one in eight did so every month.

Section six was about *Pregnancy and breastfeeding*.

The breasts start to change early in pregnancy, as we shall see on page 127, and 24 per cent of our sample noticed breast changes in the first month of pregnancy. Approximately 20 per cent noticed first changes in each of the next three months and some women claimed that they had no breast changes until the fifth, sixth or even the seventh month.

Although we had encountered many a raised eyebrow when it came to the subject of the sexual enjoyment (from the mother's point of view) of breastfeeding, we had long felt that many more women experienced sexually pleasant sensations while breastfeeding than would admit to it. This is a shame because there is no doubt from our experience that some women give up feeding because of these feelings, some even describing the sensation as 'incestuous'. We were gratified therefore to find that among our sample over half (64 per cent) said that they had found breastfeeding 'sexually pleasant' or 'sensual'. Many men worry that their partners will go off them if they are breastfeeding but exactly half of our sample said that their sexual relationship didn't change at all during breastfeeding. However, a third said that things changed for the worse and only 15 per cent said things were better. Of those whose sex lives changed at all, the biggest single change was that the man was put off the woman's breasts. We shall look at this in more detail in Chapter 4.

What women say about their breasts

It is difficult to write a book about the breast without becoming acutely aware of women's deepest feelings about this part of their anatomy. Even the words women use when talking about their breasts are interesting and revealing. Many women find the word 'breast' itself intimidating (too medical) and use 'bust' or 'boobs' instead — words that have fewer emotional overtones. Very few people in the corsetry business talk of 'breasts' to their customers. The word 'bust' has been adopted as a sort of neutral, conceptual term for the area of the chest that women hide in their bras. Unfortunately this serves to remove it even further in most women's psyches from the organs that they use for feeding and comforting babies (breasts).

What comes across most of all in listening to women talking about their breasts is their insecurity about them, and this is borne out by the massive correspondence to magazine agony aunts on the subject. Our questionnaire results helped identify some of these insecurities in more detail. To some women the very thought of talking about their breasts, except in the most 'medical' way, was revolting. Younger women by and large were more open, so perhaps there is hope for the future.

Obviously we can only give a sketchy outline, and a highly selective one at that, of the sorts of thing women say about their breasts but we hope they'll be useful to others who think they're alone with their 'funny ideas' about *their* breasts. We've tried to choose some often-repeated and representative thoughts from the thousands of women we've discussed breasts and breastfeeding with over the years.

'If a partner didn't like my breasts there would be no point in sex with him — my breasts are *me*.'

'My breasts are my most responsive point — they act as a remote control to my clitoris area.'

'I only like to wear a bra as a sexual turn-on for my man when I take it off.'

'As soon as my breasts are touched by anyone I physically shudder.

Any sexual feelings I had before completely disappear and it's a real effort for me to disguise my feelings. Obviously this puts lovemaking in danger and I just can't seem to alter the way I feel. If my breasts aren't touched I feel completely satisfied and orgasm frequently. I wonder, am I a freak? I met someone else who hated her breasts being touched so obviously I'm not the only one. PS: I breast-fed three children happily and realized that this is what breasts were really for. Obviously my poor husband has terrible problems coming to terms with my difference of views on this.'

'After breastfeeding (and even during it) my breasts became extremely potent as an erogenous zone. This effect didn't wear off and my nipples are still very erotic indeed.'

'I was fourteen when a boy first touched my breasts under my clothes . . . he was very disappointed!'

'I've had four operations for abscesses and infections. Of course, I was worried that it was cancer but the hospital weren't very understanding about my worries. As they took bits out I became worried that eventually I'd be left with no breast at all. If my condition *had* been cancer I think it would have been easier to come to terms with. It's very hard for me to accept the mess the operations have made of my breasts, especially the nipples which are very odd now.'

'I didn't realize how much women (and me in particular) had come to believe that their breasts were so important to them. Even now, though I'm not sure why, it's having an enormous effect on the relationship with my husband. Presumably this could be a factor that could result in the forming of a new relationship. Basically, although I've had all the trouble, I don't know anything about my breasts, even though my GP has been very understanding.'

'I am eighty-eight, have had several affairs before and since my husband died in 1964 but breasts are, in my opinion, greatly overrated.'

'The concept of an "ideal" breast that you talk about in your questionnaire is absolute nonsense. There's no such thing. All breasts are different, uniquely individual and are a part of the woman herself. There is no stereotype.'

'I think women worry much too much about their breasts and that this has come about mainly because of media portrayal and stereotypes. These produce insecure feelings among women.'

'I find it very extraordinary having hairy breasts. I used to cut the hairs off but now I don't bother.'

'My partner loves my breasts when I'm feeding because they're larger.'

'If anything, breastfeeding has improved my shape.'

'I found your question "What do you think of women who go without bras?" disturbing in its assumptions. Why didn't you have a question "What do you think of women who *do* wear bras?" Also I found your questionnaire automatically excluded homosexual relationships. Because of this I feel I must ask you to withdraw my questionnaire from your analysis.'

'My partner would like my breasts to be larger but he doesn't want me to use any particular method.'

'When I was breastfeeding I found it difficult to reconcile my breasts as sexual things when they were feeding implements for my son. I thought of them as his property rather than mine or my husband's. My husband, however, found it all very exciting.'

'Women with large breasts are ignored by the fashion industry thus making it difficult to buy clothes, and often I end up buying men's tops. This makes me feel abnormal and awkward.'

'I wore bras for a few years, mainly through force of habit, but gave them up when I was sixteen because they were limiting and un-comfortable.'

'I welcome your research because, as you say, the answers to the questions you're asking can't be readily found anywhere.'

'My view is that men think a woman's breast should be erect, pointed and high up on her chest, rather like an erect penis and on offer to men. They're meant to be passive and certainly not to move. I was lucky because my father thought bras were superfluous fashion items and my mother allowed me a free choice . . . An aunt of mine found my bralessness quite beyond the pale, beyond anything she had ever encountered and made no efforts to hide her reactions. She could not work out whether I was a prostitute or maybe there was something wrong with me. Her behaviour caused me great psychological distress at the time. People don't realize that a twelve-or thirteen-year-old girl is so impressionable and hasn't got the courage of a fifty-year-old. From that day to this she has not liked me . . . '

'All my boyfriends prefer me to go braless especially my present one (a professor of gynaecology!) who is positively put off by the concept of the "ideal" breast.'

'I frequently experience orgasms when my boyfriend stimulates my breasts alone. Many women will feel that this is impossible.'

'My partner is a sensitive man who has very commonsense attitudes to my breasts. I feel I am luckier than most women. He believes that breasts are naturally floppy and likes them that way.'

'If I had a baby I would definitely want to breastfeed it. This is because I feel it would be better for the child and because I would find breastfeeding a deeply satisfying experience.'

'A girl in our office has just left because (I have since learned) she couldn't bear me having better breasts than she had.'

'The thought of breastfeeding is absolutely revolting. I don't want a man being a baby to me either, sucking my breasts or anything. When I was young and my breasts were developing I hated it because I didn't want my Dad to notice; I didn't want him to look at me sexually. In fact my breasts only began to mean anything at all to me when boys started to like them but then and now I don't like them much. They embarrass me and get in the way. Frankly, if they turn a man on, OK but that's all. They do absolutely nothing for me. I'm not anti my breasts or anything but they are completely neutral for me.'

'When I was about fourteen I had a lump which became inflamed and very painful, but I was far too embarrassed to tell my mother or doctor. It disappeared overnight about a week later and I told my mother ten years later.'

'Thank you for sending me your questionnaire – it's nice to know someone's interested. I am fifteen and my breasts haven't stopped growing yet. Usually I feel happy with them but sometimes when particularly depressed I want to change them but only in the same way I'd like to change other parts of my body. I get a lot of sexual pleasure from them and they are well worth having even though I don't want any children and won't need them biologically. I also get a lot of pleasure from other women's breasts and like holding them. Incidentally, I have never worn a bra and hope I will never have to.'

'When I masturbate I often try to suck my nipples but my neck isn't flexible enough or long enough.'

'A schoolfriend of mine told me that if I didn't buy a bra I'd have trouble later on. I felt a bit scared of her so I bought one.'

'I'm only sixteen and my breasts haven't stopped growing. I've got stretch marks and I don't know if they'll go. My mum says they probably won't but I'd like them to and soon. I get a lot of pleasure from my breasts and I like other women's breasts. I don't want my breasts to get any bigger — they are already 36½.'

'If only people realized how awful it is having big breasts. Men are foul to you — you get wolf whistles from all the wrong ones. I had endless backache and neck pain and couldn't get a bra anywhere. I really felt a freak. In the end I had to have plastic surgery — life just wasn't worth living any more.'

'I find sexual spontaneity hampered during breastfeeding . . . is this what they mean by natural family planning?'

'I am very concerned about the long-term effect of going without a bra and wonder if it could harm my breasts. For example, will it build firmer muscles to support my breasts going without a bra? Or will it simply make them more heavy and saggy?'

'Breastfeeding has changed our sex life. Before I fed I wasn't really bothered about my breasts at all — in fact I had thought them rather too large. Feeding made me aware of the pleasurable sensations I *could* get from my breasts from sucking. Now my partner can turn me on this way although when I am feeding the milk turns him off. He felt he had to hold back because of his excessive closeness to his mother (he's an only child) and this prevented him from enjoying my breasts fully. This plus my episiotomy made our sexual relationship poor during breastfeeding but it is better now.'

'When a man considers only a part of my body without consideration for my personality I don't like it.'

'I'm fifty-seven and I like having my breasts kissed and I'm terribly guilty because I find it boring sometimes. My breasts are droopy but my nipples are responsive. I'm not at all "woman's lib" but just want my fellow to be happy and now that we are approaching our dotage I expect we shall continue as we are.'

'If men didn't have such a breast fetish it would be much nicer because then I could go topless especially in the summer. It makes me angry to think that women are made to feel indecent if they show their breasts. I'd like to get sun on my chest the way men do.'

'Sometimes I dream of having an orgasm while caressing another woman's breasts.'

'One of my breasts is larger than the other — I wish they were both smaller.'

'I can't bear to hear men talk about "tits" or "knockers". "Breasts" to me mean something lovely, full, rounded and sensual.'

'My breasts are at the very centre of my lovemaking – without them I wouldn't be me.'

CHAPTER 2

What breasts are and what they do

Men and women are members of a group of animals called mammals, all of which are characterized by the presence of milk-secreting glands or mammary glands. The word 'breasts' is used only to describe human mammary glands, not those of other mammals.

The size, number and shape of mammary glands vary from species to species and under normal circumstances the gland becomes functional only in the female, even though mammary tissue is present in both sexes (except in male marsupials). In most species the glands are paired. Humans and the goat have two, and the pig fourteen to eighteen, for example. The position of the glands is also very variable. In the rodent, dog, pig and rabbit they are situated along the chest and abdomen; in humans, bats and elephants they are on the chest; in ruminants (animals that chew the cud) they are in the groin; in the whale, on the abdomen; and in the coypu, on the back.

The shapes of mammary glands are just about as varied too. In rats and mice they are flat sheets of tissue around the body wall; in the rabbit and monkey they are flat and circular; and in ruminants (for example, cows and goats) pairs lie closely together to form an udder. All mammals except the monotremes – the group of Australian mammals that includes the echidnas (spiny anteaters) and the platypus – have a nipple on the tip of each gland.

In spite of all these external differences, the interior structure of mammary glands, whatever the species, is remarkably constant. Glandular tissue and ducts lie within supporting tissue and even the most careful electron microscopy reveals few differences in the milk-producing cells from species to species.

In humans, just as in other mammals, the breasts develop from specialized structures in the skin. In fact, the breast is a sort of specialized sweat gland. At about the fifth or sixth week of fetal life a number of papillae develop along two 'milk-lines' or ridges that run from the groins to the armpits. This happens both in males and females. By the ninth week most of the line on each side has disappeared leaving only one papilla (nipple) on each side in the chest

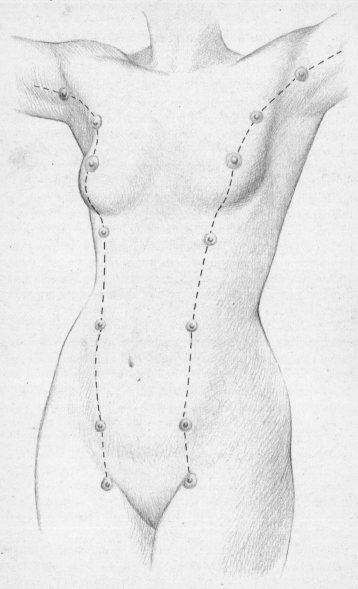

A schematic drawing to show the milk lines. Extra nipples (and theoretically breasts) can occur anywhere along these lines.

area. By the end of the third month skin cells have formed a nipple bud and duct tissue starts forming. Lactiferous (milk) ducts begin to form and open on to the nipple via a lactiferous sinus (collecting reservoir) which lies just under the nipple. Pigment is deposited around the nipple to form the areola.

In humans the breasts are undeveloped at birth and only develop at puberty when there is a deposition of fat and connective tissue and a proliferation of milk ducts. The milk-producing cells (already present at birth) only develop in any major way during pregnancy.

Because of this type of development several abnormalities can occur. Extra breast tissue or nipples can occur anywhere along the milk line if it hasn't been re-absorbed as usual, whereas excessive re-absorption can mean there is no nipple or breast on the affected side. The commonest abnormality of development by far is the presence of extra nipples – and these, strange as it may seem, are more common in men (see page 235).

During childhood there is very little activity in the breast but at puberty the hypothalamus (a specialized part of the brain) 'turns on' the production of several hormones that initiate breast and ovarian function. Under the influence of these hormones the breasts grow at a rate which outstrips the growth of the rest of the body. This growth of

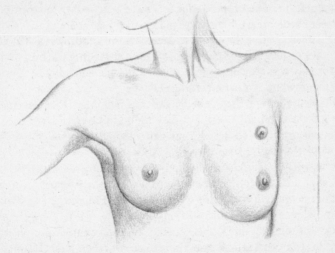

An extra nipple like this can occur anywhere along the milk line. They are seen in men too.

the breasts (doctors call it the thelarche) is usually the first sign of puberty. Before a balance is produced between ovarian and pituitary hormones, a girl has cycles that are not accompanied by ovulation (as is the case in a mature woman). At this stage the breast is mainly under the influence of oestrogens. The duct system elongates and branches and fat deposition goes ahead apace. Once the girl starts to ovulate, progesterone is added to the hormonal mix and further breast changes occur.

There are several well-defined stages in the development of young girls' breasts. In the first stage there is pre-adolescent elevation of the nipple only, no glandular tissue and no areolar pigmentation. Except for the nipple the breast doesn't project from the chest wall.

Stage two of the development involves the growth of areolar and glandular tissue. The nipple and the breast now project as a single mound from the chest wall. The average time for this to occur in white girls in the West is about the age of eleven.

Stage three is that at which more glandular tissue is formed and the areolae become enlarged and pigmented. The contours of the breast and nipple remain in one plane. This happens on average around the age of twelve.

During stage four there is further breast enlargement and nipple pigmentation. The nipple and areola form a secondary mound above the rest of the breast. This takes place on average at about thirteen.

During stage five the nipple and areola no longer project as a mound but have returned to be part of the smooth contour of the breast. The breast may still grow in volume a little after this until about the age of seventeen when it is usually full size.

There are several disease states, most of them rare, that can change this developmental pattern but they need not be considered here. If ever you are worried about your daughter's development put your mind at rest by discussing it with your doctor.

The one thing that is especially important to remember is that breast size has absolutely nothing to do with their sexual or breast-feeding potential. Many girls worry that if their breasts are small their partners may be less likely to enjoy them sexually. Women with breasts of all sizes enjoy their breasts as erotic centres and whether they do so or not has little or nothing to do with their size. Of course, a girl (or a mature woman for that matter) who feels insecure and unhappy with her breasts may behave in a way which puts men off her

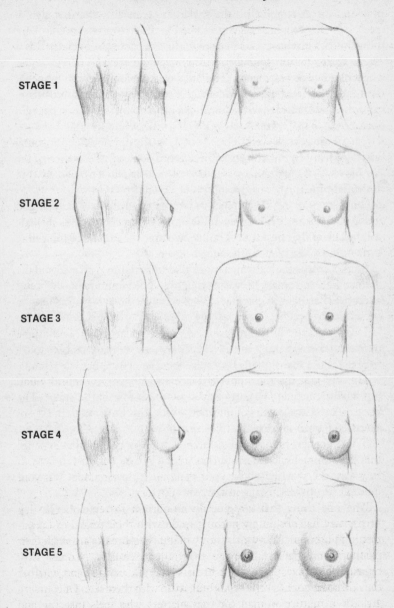

STAGE 1

STAGE 2

STAGE 3

STAGE 4

STAGE 5

The development of the breast during puberty.

breasts. In this way she produces exactly the sort of response she so fears. The opposite occurs with girls who are proud of and at ease with their breasts because their behaviour encourages men to enjoy them and so they get more pleasure out of them themselves. A mother has a real responsibility to ensure that her daughters grow up at ease with their breasts, not feeling guilty or inferior about them. This can be especially difficult because many teenage girls are so mixed up and ambivalent about their sexuality that it's difficult for a parent to know what to do for the best.

Let's look now at the adult female breast.

The breasts lie on the chest wall over two muscles that move the arm — the pectoral muscles. The substance of the breasts lies on a roughly circular base the top of which is at the level of the second or third rib and the bottom at the fifth or sixth rib. However, many women have an axillary tail of breast tissue that extends up into the armpit and some women's breasts cover a much wider area of the chest wall than just described.

The mature female breast is roughly conical in shape but considerable changes take place as the breast ages, the tendency being for the tissues to become looser and the breasts to sag and become flatter. This happens because fat is lost and not because the amount of glandular tissue is very much less. Also, as a woman ages the connective tissues that support the breast weaken. The skin of the breasts is like that anywhere else on the body but produces unsightly scars very easily when cut. This can be almost totally avoided if any incision made follows the natural skin lines which run in concentric circles around the nipple and areola. The skin of the nipple and areola has no hair but around the areola some women have a number of hair follicles, some of which produce quite long hairs. Hair over the rest of the breast is very fine like that on the rest of a woman's body. For what to do about unsightly hairs around the areola, see page 104.

The skin of the breast has the same type of nerve supply as that of the rest of the body but the nipple has erogenous (sexually arousable) tissue that is supplied with many nerves. Erotic stimulation of the nipples is a potent source of arousal for most women though only about half of all women claim their nipples are important to them sexually. The skin of the areola is the most sensitive part of the breast in a non-aroused, non-pregnant woman and that of the nipple the least sensitive to pain and other stimuli. Larger breasts are usually less sensitive to stimuli than are smaller ones, and among women with small or moderately sized breasts those who have been pregnant have greater sensation in their nipples and areolae than do other women.

On the top of the cone of breast tissue is the *nipple* surrounded by a darker area of the skin called the *areola*. The nipple usually projects from the surface of the areola a little (the amount varies enormously, even in any one woman) and becomes more obvious when it is cold, on rubbing against clothes, on removal of a bra, when it is stimulated sexually and during the breastfeeding months, especially when the baby is actually at the breast. The nipple becomes larger because it contains many small muscle fibres that can contract to make it erect. During sexual stimulation and during lactation (especially as the let-down reflex works) there is also a considerable local increase in blood flow and this makes the whole breast, including the nipple, swell considerably. Special sweat glands are present on the areolar skin where they appear as tiny protuberances called Montgomery's tubercles. These enlarge in pregnancy in some women (see page 127). Recent research has shown that these tubercles are exactly like miniature breasts in their structure and function. Indeed, in some women they become functional during lactation.

Nipples vary greatly in shape and size. The tip of the nipple is pockmarked by fifteen to twenty deep crevices which are usually filled with horny plugs. Most nipples are cylindrical in shape but some are fissured, some conical, some mushroom-shaped, some inverted (flat or pushed inwards) and others like a mulberry. (See page 42).

The colour of the nipple and areola varies from woman to woman according to the type of complexion she has and also alters with pregnancy. As a general rule, red-haired women have very pale pink areolae, fair-haired women slightly darker pink, and then the areola becomes gradually darker as a woman's complexion darkens – black women have nearly black areolae. All women's areolae and nipples become slightly (or sometimes very much) darker during pregnancy and never return to their original state completely. They do not, however, continue to darken with each successive pregnancy.

So much for the external appearance of the breast; now to the internal structure.

Inside each breast there are about twenty *lobes*, each divided off from the other by compartments of connective tissue. The breasts rely greatly on this connective and fibrous tissue 'skeleton' for their

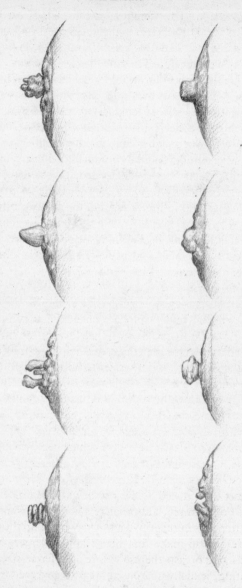

Some normal variations of nipple shape.

support and shape. The weight of the breasts is carried by these fibrous bands that are attached to the upper chest wall and to the skin of the breasts. These same suspensory ligaments, as they are called, are extremely well developed in some species. The cow, for example, needs formidable support for its udder which can weigh 40 kg (90 lb) or more! Each lobe has its own milk *duct* which opens at the nipple. Just underneath the surface each duct expands to form a cone-shaped area in which milk collects just before it is released from the nipple. Each of the twenty or so lobes contains vast numbers of *lobules*, each containing large numbers of milk-producing cells surrounding a small milk-collecting duct. So the whole structure of the breast's milk-producing system looks rather like a complex collection of grapes with the grapes lying deep in the breast and the stalks coming out at the nipple.

During lactation milk is constantly being produced by the milk-producing cells and some is pushed along the ducts to the reservoirs collecting beneath the nipples ready for the baby to drink at the beginning of a feed.

In between all these glandular structures and their ducts there are fat, nerves, arteries, veins, lymphatic channels and connective tissue. There is no muscle in the breast at all (except for tiny bundles of muscle in and around the milk ducts that help expel milk and others in the nipple that erect it), so any effort to improve the breast aimed at 'improving muscle tone' is a complete waste of time. Such exercises can *apparently* improve breast size because they build up the chest muscles underlying the breast, which is then pushed forward by the larger muscles.

Many women's breasts are of unequal size, though not very obviously so. Others have breasts of very different sizes indeed and may seek the help of a plastic surgeon (see page 210). Sometimes the 'larger' breast is produced by the muscle underneath being used very frequently. For example, a librarian or a housewife who uses one arm repeatedly to perform repetitive tasks may build up the chest muscle on that side and so make that breast appear larger. More usually though the actual breasts themselves are of different sizes. The size of a non-lactating, sexually unaroused breast is governed by two things: first, the amount of fat and second, the amount of glandular tissue it contains. Fatter women tend to have larger breasts than do thinner ones and large, well-developed breasts by and large also contain more

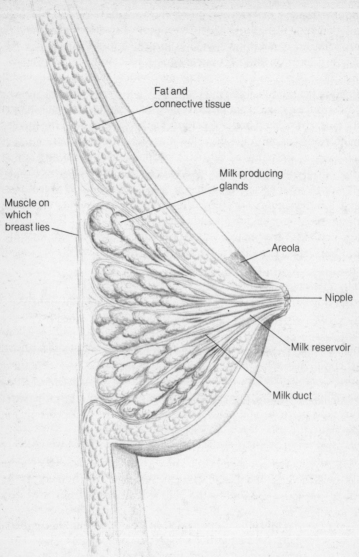

Fat and
connective tissue

Milk producing
glands

Muscle on
which
breast lies

Areola

Nipple

Milk reservoir

Milk duct

A schematic section through a breast to show its internal structure. For a description of the parts see page 43.

glandular tissue. This does not, however, mean that a woman who has small breasts will be unlikely to be able to breastfeed. Even very small-breasted women have enough glandular tissue to be able to produce plenty of milk. The average non-lactating breast weighs about 200 g (7 oz) and the lactating one about 500 g (17 oz), though these figures vary considerably.

Not only can one woman have breasts of unequal size but the variations in size and actual position of the breasts are very great. Some women are naturally very 'low-breasted' and some very 'high'. This is almost certainly an inherited phenomenon and there is little one can do about it. A bra will tend to bring the 'low-slung' woman's breasts into what society considers a 'good' position (see page 229). The size and position of the nipple on the breast are also very variable. Some women's nipples are placed not at the tip of the cone but slightly below and this gives an appearance of sagging even though there is none. The areola can vary in diameter too from 3 cm to 10 cm (1 to 4 inches) and still be perfectly normal.

The shape, size, position, skin colouring and so on of the breasts are usually inherited so there is little one can do about what nature gives a woman. It's important to remember that a girl may not inherit her breast characteristics from her mother but from her father. This explains how it is that girls often don't have breasts like their mothers'. This same explanation also accounts for the fact that mothers and daughters often have very different times of breast development. Girls develop breasts at very different ages anyway. White girls living in temperate climates tend to develop breasts a year or two earlier than others and normal breast growth can occur at any time from seven or eight until fourteen or fifteen. A girl who hasn't started developing by fourteen or fifteen will probably want to seek medical advice, though usually nothing at all will need to be done. In most white girls the breasts have reached their full size by about the age of seventeen.

A woman's weight affects her breasts quite considerably. A woman who is overweight for a long time will stretch not only the connective tissue beneath the skin but also the fibrous tissue 'walls' that make up the compartments of the breast and attach it to the skin and the upper chest wall. When this woman then loses weight she'll have stretch marks which are very difficult (if not impossible) to remove. Some young girls who are fat complain that their breasts are too small, when in reality the fat all around the chest wall masks the true size of their breasts. Having overweight breasts doesn't alter their biological function including their ability to produce milk in any way so the problems are nearly all aesthetic. A well-fitting bra can help the woman who has obese breasts but this will, of course, do nothing to *cure* the condition.

Some women are concerned because as they put on weight their areolae seem to get bigger. This occurs purely because of the stretching of the skin. The areolae go back to normal size once the weight is lost. Incidentally, no amount of massage or any other non-surgical therapy will reduce the size of a breast with too much fat in it. Most plastic surgeons will want a woman to slim before they undertake to reduce a very obese breast because if the woman slims after the operation the result can be a very strange appearance.

What breasts do

Basically, as we have seen, the breast is a kind of super-specialized sweat gland and just like any other sweat gland it produces secretions all the time. In our society, for the majority of a woman's life her breasts are not lactating (producing milk) but they nevertheless produce tiny amounts of normal secretions. These can be expressed from the nipples of many women and appear spontaneously in others. If ever this natural secretion amounts to more than a drop or two at a time it's sensible to see a doctor. For a further discussion of nipple discharge, see page 113.

The breasts of human females have two main functions. First and foremost they are sexual signals of femaleness and second, they produce milk for the young. In our society, in which bottle feeding is the norm, the second function has become very unimportant, so leaving the breasts to be seen as purely sexual organs by most women. We shall look at the breast as a sex organ in Chapter 4, so let's look here at the other main function of the breasts – the production of milk to nourish the young.

Milk production by the glandular tissue of the breast occurs under the influence of several hormones including prolactin, growth hormone, thyroid hormones, corticosteroids and insulin. Each milk gland is surrounded by a fine network of blood vessels which takes these hormones to the cells. The blood supply also produces the materials from which milk is actively made by the cells.

Prolactin is the main milk-producing hormone and appears in the blood from the eighth week of pregnancy onwards, reaching its peak at the birth of the baby. It does not produce milk in any volume during pregnancy because the high levels of placental oestrogen in the woman's body act as a brake on its milk-producing effects. With the loss of the placenta after birth, oestrogen levels fall and the breasts start producing milk. In our society with its rigid breastfeeding schedules this usually occurs during the second to fourth days after birth but it can be accelerated by encouraging the baby to suck at the breast very frequently throughout the day and night right from the time of birth.

The milk supply usually builds up slowly over several days but in some women it comes in a deluge. The way to cope with this latter situation is to allow the baby to suck very frequently so as to keep the breasts comfortable and unengorged (for more details, see page 67).

Prolactin, then, 'turns on the taps'. During lactation it is produced by the pituitary gland at the base of the brain in response to nipple stimulation which in turn sends nervous messages to the pituitary. The holding and squeezing of the nipple and areola by the baby's mouth stimulates the nervous pathways to increase the milk supply, so the more the baby stimulates the nipple, the more milk is made.

As milk is produced by the milk glands in between feeds some of it passes into the milk ducts and thence to the reservoirs under the areolae. These reservoirs can store up to a third of the milk for the next feed ready for the baby as soon as he wants it. This milk, known as *foremilk*, is low in fat and thus in calories. Every woman produces milk after birth and so will have some foremilk but the bulk of the milk a baby needs (the other two-thirds of its feed) is only supplied if a particular nervous reflex called the *let-down reflex* is activiated.

After a feed the milk-producing cells gradually distend with milk as more is formed. This fullness produces a lumpiness in the breasts of some women. The milk is forced into the ducts very quickly by the contraction of the muscle cells surrounding each milk gland. When this happens the milk is said to have been 'let-down'. This reflex must operate if the baby is to get the milk held in the glands (as opposed to that stored in the reservoirs under the nipple). When this let-down occurs milk spurts from the ducts with such force that it can spray some distance from the nipples. This often occurs in a series of spurts from several ducts at once.

Milk produced by the let-down reflex is called *hindmilk* and forms the bulk of a feed, as we have seen. This milk is rich in fat and therefore in calories and without it the baby will not get enough nourishment to thrive. Foremilk contains 1.5 calories/ounce and hindmilk 30 calories/ounce. The reason that many women fail to breastfeed is that their let-down reflex doesn't work. It is a finely balanced mechanism (as any dairy farmer will confirm) especially in the early weeks after birth when many external factors can inhibit it. When people talk about the 'establishment' of breast-feeding they are really talking about the establishment of a satisfactory, reliable and effective let-down reflex.

The main factor involved in this reflex is nipple stimulation. This is the same stimulus that produces prolactin release. But another hormone is required for the operation of the let-down reflex – oxytocin. This is the substance that makes the muscle cells around the milk glands contract and push the milk into the ducts, and forces the milk out – sometimes in sprays or jets – from the nipple. The time taken for the let-down reflex to work varies from woman to woman and even within any one woman it can vary from day to day according to her surroundings, her emotional state and several other factors. Once a baby is put to the breast the let-down takes a minimum of thirty to fifty seconds to work but it often takes longer – two to three minutes or more is not uncommon.

This means that a hungry baby may have finished all the foremilk before the hindmilk is available and this can make him frustrated. Such frustration can so worry the inexperienced mother that she doesn't let down her milk at all.

Nipple stimulation isn't the only way that the let-down reflex can be triggered. The sight or sound of a woman's baby (or even someone else's) can suddenly let down her milk, especially if it's some time since the last feed. Some women find that as they prepare to feed they let down in anticipation, the routine has so conditioned their natural reflexes. Even thinking about a baby can trigger the let-down.

As well as causing the let-down, oxytocin has other effects. The uterus is sensitive to it and may contract when the blood levels of oxytocin are raised. Such uterine contractions are rhythmical and are the cause of the 'after pains' some mothers experience while feeding in the early days. Some women also find that their breasts tingle or feel tense. The let-down is usually a pleasant feeling though and has been described as 'something between a sneeze and an orgasm'. We will see in Chapter 4 that orgasms, breastfeeding and childbirth are all basically similar in many ways and that the pleasurable nature of them all is brought about by the hormone oxytocin. Because of this, one leading US researcher in this field has called it the 'love hormone'.

As the milk is let down, the skin of the breasts becomes warmer and this, together with the contraction of the womb and the leaking from the breasts, is a very good sign that the let-down is working well. Some mothers have none of these signs yet let-down very well. Women vary a lot in their experience of the let-down, even from baby to baby – the description we have given may not be typical for you.

So this then is the way in which the breasts produce and deliver milk. It's interesting that the milk yield in humans and, indeed, in other mammals, is related to body weight. Also, related to the weight of milk-producing tissue, the yield per gramme of tissue in most species is exactly the same. One gramme of tissue usually produces about 1 gramme of milk. The frequency of suckling varies greatly from species to species, though. Rats nurse their young fifty to eighty times a day while at the other end of the scale the tree shrew visits her young only once every forty-eight hours. We shall see how important nursing frequency is for human babies in the chapter on breastfeeding (see page 52).

As the average woman in the Western world has only two babies, the milk-producing ability of her breasts is little used. Cyclical changes, however, occur *every* month in the breast and because they occur many hundreds of times in a woman's reproductive life we shall look at them here.

During the reproductive years the breasts undergo cyclical changes with a woman's monthly cycle. In the few days before a period (menstruation) the breasts swell and become firmer, more nodular and, in some women, tender to the touch. Quite a lot is now known about breast sensitivity at various times in a woman's life, and it has been shown that it is greatest at ovulation (half-way through the cycle) and at menstruation. The mid-cycle ovulatory peak is absent in women taking the Pill.

These monthly breast changes occur as a prelude to a possible pregnancy but if this doesn't occur the breasts return to their normal size by the third or fourth day of menstruation. The fullness of the breasts in the pre-menstrual stage is caused by a retention of fluid and by some increased cellular activity too. Certainly the blood flow to the breasts is greatly increased pre-menstrually and most women have an increased breast volume of about 100 ml (3.5 fl. oz) – up to 30 per cent – at this time. Women on the Pill seem to experience less breast swelling at this time – 66 ml (2.3 fl. oz) – on average. Because all these changes alter the 'feel' of the breast it is not wise to examine for lumps at this time because the feel is so atypical of the resting breast. A real lump will be present at all the phases of the monthly cycle but transitory 'false' lumps can often be felt pre-menstrually and can cause unnecessary concern.

We shall see how the breast changes during pregnancy in Chapter 6.

From the time childbearing ceases most women have a twenty-year span of menstrual cycles until the menopause, and we saw in Chapter 1 that this might well have deleterious effects. As the menopause approaches the breasts begin to involute. As ovarian function wanes around the menopause these are two fairly distinct phases of this involution. The first occurs between thirty-five and forty-five during which there is a moderate decrease in glandular tissue. The menopausal or senile phase starts at about forty-five and progresses until about seventy-five. The amount of glandular tissue falls significantly and fat deposition increases, as does connective tissue. The breasts become flatter and more pendulous, their skin wrinkles and they do not, of course, undergo cyclical changes. Many women, however, still get sexual pleasure from their breasts and their nipples are still erogenous centres for them.

So throughout a woman's life her breasts are ever-changing, reflecting her underlying hormonal patterns, her childbearing and her breastfeeding. The sensible woman gets to know her breasts intimately and shares this knowledge with her partner so that both understand the many facets of her breasts in health and disease. In this way both of them get maximum pleasure from them over the years and any abnormalities are detected and treated without delay. For more details about what you and your partner can do at a monthly examination, see page 134.

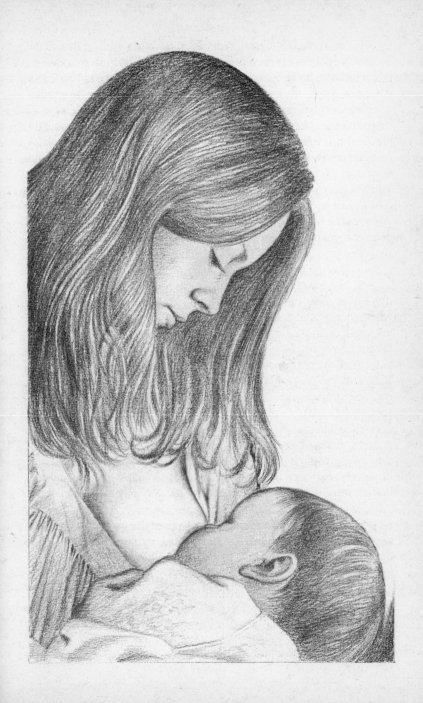

CHAPTER 3

Breastfeeding

Introduction

Breastfeeding, for millions of years the normal and virtually the only way to feed a baby, reached an all-time low in the middle of this century in the Western world. The fashionable way to feed babies in the USA, Australia, New Zealand, South Africa, Great Britain and most of Europe was to bottle-feed them with cows' milk, usually modified in one way or another. Today there is an enormous resurgence of interest in breastfeeding in these countries but even so most babies have more cows' milk than breast milk.

This obsession with bottle-feeding arose for several reasons, one of them being that modern techniques of milk production and the preparation and giving of feeds made artificial feeding with modified cows' milk safer than it had previously been. Spurred on by the enormous advertising expenditure of the babymilk companies together with a plethora of 'experts' proclaiming that cows' milk formula was as good as breast milk for babies, bottle-feeding soon became the norm.

It is no accident that the dairying economies have led the rest of the world into bottle-feeding with cows' milk. These countries and their governments have a vested interest in encouraging the consumption of cows' milk, for obvious reasons. Because cows' milk is a relatively cheap source of protein and contains many other nutrients as well, nutritionists have stressed repeatedly the 'needs' of everyone, especially pregnant mothers, babies and children, for such milk, and the public has come to assume that it is not only essential for health but also that it has semi-magical properties.

The opposite is, in fact, true. Cows' milk is not only completely nonessential but can be positively harmful to some people. One researcher has called the vast swing to the bottle-feeding of babies with cows' milk this century 'the largest uncontrolled medical trial ever carried out in the history of mankind'. In recent years not only has more and more evidence come to light on the disadvantages of cows' milk to babies as far as their immediate and long-term health goes, but it is also becoming clear that our over-emphasis on cows' milk may harm adults too.

The swing back to breastfeeding is occurring for a variety of reasons. Doctors and nurses like to tell themselves it is because of their health education: telling the public of the advantages of breast milk to babies in the light of recent medical research. In reality it probably has more to do with the emergence of the women's liberation movement, strange though that may at first seem. As women have become increasingly confident in themselves and their abilities, more liberated sexually and less afraid of expressing their sexuality in childbearing and breastfeeding, and more aware of taking care of their bodies, some have realized that they were missing out on one of the wonderful experiences available to them. Added to that, the public as a whole is interested in a return to a more natural way of life and understands that each individual can do a tremendous amount to improve his health.

Unfortunately, when women wanted to start breastfeeding again, they discovered to their bitter dismay that they couldn't do it! Health professionals had lost their passed-down skills of teaching and helping women to breastfeed through lack of practice, and the older generation of women – relatives, neighbours, friends and so on – had probably bottle-fed their babies and were also in no position to support and encourage the young mothers. Because of the ready availability of cows' milk formulae, there was no great incentive to breastfeed. Whereas a century or so ago the only chance of survival for a baby whose mother couldn't breastfeed was for it to be breast-fed by another woman, today that baby can be put on the bottle at once. The picture today is that more and more women are attempting to breast-feed but that large numbers give up before they really want to stop.

We can all help reverse this trend towards breastfeeding failure in society. Health professionals can seek out and arrange better training for themselves, so that instead of learning breastfeeding advice based on bottle-feeding or old wives' tales, they in fact learn how breast-feeding works and how to help mothers overcome problems. The public can help breastfeeding mothers by being more accepting of women actually doing it, rather than paying lip service to the idea that mothers should breastfeed then having fits of embarrassment if they see it happening. Women can help themselves by learning about breastfeeding and by asking for the help of the people who really know what they are doing in this area. Mother-to-mother support groups are invaluable for general advice and encouragement and have done much to increase the numbers of mothers successfully breastfeeding. The media too can help by talking about breastfeeding and by showing it happening, instead of sticking a bottle in any baby's mouth that happens to be in a photograph or on television.

Mothering

Alongside the unpopularity of breastfeeding has gone the down-grading of motherhood in society's eyes. This is an extremely complex subject, as any sociologist knows, and we can only talk about a few factors here. Perhaps one of the most interesting is that so many countries are experiencing a population explosion and it is in their interests to encourage women to have fewer babies. The result is that today's women are educated to think of themselves as wage-earners and career women rather than as wives and mothers and the majority of women spend most of their lives working rather than rearing children. Childbearing is condensed into a few years. There are fewer children in each family and they are born close together. Children are sent out to day nursery, playgroup, nursery school and school proper as early as possible, and the mother seeks fulfilment in her role at work rather than within her family. When she is at home with babies, there is little support for her and she is likely to be alone a lot, so depression and overtiredness all too easily overwhelm her and as a result she often gets little enjoyment out of her children.

What would be lovely to see — and is happening in some areas — is the development of an awareness of motherhood as being extremely important not only for society as a whole but also for each individual mother and child. Alongside this, breastfeeding — the natural and normal thing to do — would be accepted, welcomed and encouraged, and health professionals and the public together could forget their anxieties about routines and schedules and getting children away from their mothers as quickly as possible, and could concentrate instead on helping mothers relax and enjoy their babies. Along with this general relaxation in attitudes and a desire for the best possible mothering for babies would automatically come more successful breastfeeding — breastfeeding for as long as the mother and her baby want.

Some statistics

Just to bring home what is actually happening in the UK, it's interesting to look at the last large national survey that was carried out by the Department of Health and Social Security in 1975. They studied well over two thousand mothers and looked at their attitudes to and practice of infant feeding. ['Infant Feeding 1975: Attitudes and Practice in England and Wales', (HMSO 1978)]. The following table is compiled from various figures given in their report.

Percentage of women breast or bottle feeding at different times after birth

| | Breast feeding (%) | | Bottle feeding (%) |
	Fully	Partially	
Birth	51	–	49
2 weeks	14	35	51
6 weeks	4	24	72
4 months	1	13	86
6 months	–	9	91

Although one in two women starts off breastfeeding, fewer than one in four of these mothers is still fully breastfeeding at two weeks. By six weeks only one in two of them are giving any breast milk at all, and only 4 per cent of all mothers are fully breastfeeding. By four months fewer than 1 per cent are fully breastfeeding, and only one in four of the mothers who started off breastfeeding are still giving any breast milk at all.

'So what?' we can hear you say. Well, quite apart from the unhappiness of those mothers who would have liked to have gone on breastfeeding but couldn't, expert opinion is unanimous that it is best to breastfeed for a minimum of two weeks and preferably for four to six months. Clearly we have been nowhere near achieving this, though a new study (currently under way) seems to suggest that things are gradually improving.

How breastfeeding works

We shall see how the breasts change during adolescence and in pregnancy (see pages 123 and 127 respectively), and we've already talked about the production of breast milk and how it gets to the baby (see page 46. No one knows for sure what percentage of women in any particular society are genetically incapable of producing enough milk to nourish a baby (given good health and nourishment themselves) but it seems likely that almost every women can do so if she knows what to do. Many women find that their breastfeeding experience is different with different babies. Unfortunately, the women who produce a lot of milk regardless of how often their babies feed are the very ones who go around telling other women how their babies only have five or six feeds a day and sleep through the night from a few weeks old. Most women cannot breastfeed successfully like this without their milk sooner or later drying up, leaving an unhappy and hungry baby in the meantime.

Research into the supply of breast milk has been very inadequate until fairly recently and has always centred on the first week or so of the baby's life. However, what there is has backed up the experience of breastfeeding mothers by underlining the fact that far more frequent feeds than are generally advised encourage the mother's milk to come in sooner after the birth of her baby and that this is more likely to lead to successful breastfeeding. Similarly, breast feeds which are unrestricted in length are more likely to lead to successful breast-feeding. What breastfeeding mothers say from their cumulative years of experience is that the more often and the longer they let their babies stay at the breast, the more milk there is available.

Instead of agreeing to the outdated advice still given by some hospitals of feeding babies four-hourly (or even 'three or four hourly') for ten minutes a side (and for even shorter times in the first few days), and infrequently or not at all at night, we should remember that the human baby is what biologists call a continuous contact species of animal. If allowed free access to the mother's breast most babies will suckle (suck or simply hold the breast in their mouths) very frequently indeed throughout the day and night. This is what nature intended and it's quite clear that this is what babies like: babies allowed to do this virtually never cry and their mothers nearly always have plenty of milk, provided they are healthy and well nourished themselves.

The contents of breast milk

Just as the blood from different species of mammals is different, so also is their milk. The basic groups of substances present are similar in each milk, but the proportions of each group vary tremendously and the individual groups may be made up of whole families of substances which differ both in type and proportion from species to species. Over the course of evolution, each mammal's milk has become adapted to the needs of its own young. Different animals have different rates of growth, different body make-ups, different diseases and different types of digestive tract, so it's not surprising that their milks are so different. Though we have chosen cows' milk to give as a substitute for breast milk to our babies, we could have chosen the milk of any mammal, provided we then modified it so that the proportions of its main groups of ingredients roughly matched those of breast milk. One thing we have learned – at some cost to babies' lives and health – is that however we change cows' milk, it can never be the same as, or as good as, breast milk.

Breast milk contains the following main groups of substances: water, proteins, fats, carbohydrates, minerals, vitamins, anti-infective substances, enzymes and hormones. It also contains traces of many other things present in the mother's blood, including food breakdown products she has eaten, drugs she is taking and various environmental pollutants. Let's look at each in turn.

Water: All the other contents of milk are dissolved or suspended in water, which provides all the liquid a baby needs. In a hot climate, the breastfeeding mother needs to drink more rather than give the baby extra water by bottle. Water is essential for life and a shortage can cause dehydration, cell damage and eventually death. The reason that many maternity hospitals give newborn breast-fed babies water and cows' milk formula by bottle is to provide them with sufficient liquid so that they don't become dehydrated. However, if the mother gives frequent feeds which are not restricted in length, from birth onwards, there is no reason why she should not supply all the milk – and thus the water – her baby needs.

Proteins: Human milk is a low-protein milk. This corresponds with the fact that human babies grow very slowly compared with the young of many mammals. Unmodified cows' milk has nearly three times as much protein. Both milks contain curd protein (casein) and whey proteins (lactalbumin and lactoglobulin) but cows' milk contains six times as much casein. This is why unmodified cows' milk is relatively indigestible. Breast milk is digested far quicker even than modified cows' milk, which helps explain why babies need frequent feeds when they are breast-fed. Because the protein in breast milk is so well digested and absorbed by the baby, there is little wastage and the baby needs correspondingly less milk compared with the bottle-fed baby. Besides proteins, breast milk contains specific patterns of amino acids and nucleotides which differ a lot from those in cows' milk.

Fats: Breast milk contains a relatively high proportion of unsaturated fats and — interestingly — large amounts of cholesterol. It also contains lipase, a fat-splitting enzyme also present in the baby's intestine. It is thought that the characteristic pattern of fatty acids in breast milk fat has developed so as to supply exactly what the human infant needs for the growth of many of its tissues but especially for its brain and nerves.

Carbohydrates: Lactose is present in relatively large amounts in breast milk, which explains its sweet taste. Glucose and some other sugars are also present, as is another carbohydrate — the bifidus factor — which is an important anti-infective factor.

Minerals: Breast milk has only a quarter of the total mineral content of cows' milk and while cows' milk formulae all have artificially reduced levels of minerals, it is at present impossible safely to lower the levels to those of breast milk. Sodium is one mineral which is present even in modified cows' milk in much higher amounts than in breast milk. A bottle-fed baby who is relatively dehydrated (because of a fever, vomiting or diarrhoea) can quickly build up levels of sodium which are far too high and can be life-threatening, especially if the feeds are made up too concentrated. A breast-fed baby on the other hand is quite safe, provided he is drinking enough breast milk. Calcium, phosphorus, copper, zinc, magnesium and iron are other important minerals present in proportions relatively different from those in cows' milk. The iron in breast milk is much better absorbed than that in cows' milk.

Vitamins: Breast milk contains different proportions of various vitamins compared with cows' milk formulae. In general, if a breastfeeding mother is well-nourished and has enough vitamin D-producing sunshine on her skin, there is no evidence that her baby needs any vitamin supplements.

Anti-infective substances and enzymes: Highly specialized proteins called immunoglobulins carry antibodies against various infectious bacterial or viral diseases which the mother has had or has been immunized against. Colostrum (the earliest type of breast milk) contains relatively very large amounts of these. Later in infancy the baby will produce his own antibodies in response to infection but at first he relies on those in breast milk. Antibodies in cows' milk are for various reasons ineffective for human babies. Besides antibodies the very proportions of substances in breast milk, together with the bifidus factor, lactoferrin, lysozyme, complement, anti-staphylococcal factor, hydrogen peroxide, lactoperoxidase, live cells, interferon and other anti-viral substances, all help combat infection from bacteria, viruses and fungi in the breast-fed baby.

Hormones: Comparatively little is known as yet about the role of the hormones found in breast milk but it is just possible that they may have an important bearing of the development of the breast-fed baby.

How breast milk changes

The composition of breast milk, unlike that of cows' milk formula, varies not only according to the length of time after birth (changing from colostrum − the early milk − to mature milk, and then to regression milk as weaning progresses), but also according to the time of day (when it is influenced by differing levels of hormones and other chemicals in the mother's blood, and also by the nature of and the time since the last meal the mother had), and according to the degree of emptying of the breast during a feed. Interestingly enough, mothers who have had pre-term (premature) babies temporarily produce milk of a different composition from that of mothers of full-term babies. This milk contains more protein, sodium and chloride and less lactose, and is thus tailor-made for the specific needs of the pre-term baby.

Why breast milk is best for babies

We've seen from a brief look at the composition of human milk that it contains substances in unique amounts and proportions compared with other mammalian milks, modified or not. In terms of *nourishment* it is the only milk that has been developed over millions of years of evolution specifically for the needs of human babies.

From the *growth* point of view, it seems that the contents of breast milk from a well-nourished mother are perfectly geared to the optimum rate of growth of her baby. Although breast-fed babies can get fat, this fat seems to be lost more easily later, compared with that in children who were bottle-fed. There is some reason to suppose that fat babies are at some advantage in that they have fat stores to draw on in times of illness.

There is no doubt that even in the West with its high standards of sanitation, breast-fed babies suffer from fewer *infections*, for example gastro-enteritis, respiratory syncitial virus infections and other respiratory infections. In the Third World, with contaminated water supplies, lack of sterilizing facilities, inadequate knowledge about hygiene and insufficient money to buy enough cows' milk formula powder, bottle-fed babies are at a very real risk of dying from infections, especially gastro-enteritis. Breastfeeding, particularly if the mother has enough to eat, gives the baby a good chance of living and growing up healthily. Some milk formula companies have marketed cows' milk formulae in the Third World with apparently no thought as to the potential death warrants they are handing out with each tin of milk powder.

It's interesting that it is *exclusive* breastfeeding that is most valuable for the baby. Even one feed of bottle milk can temporarily make a baby more prone to infection.

Bottle-fed babies are seven times as likely to develop *eczema* as are breast-fed babies! One survey showed that as many as one in twenty bottle-fed babies suffer from this sometimes very distressing disease. If a baby is partly breast-and partly bottle-fed, he is still twice as likely to get eczema as if he were fully breast-fed. The likelihood of developing eczema in a bottle-fed child from an 'allergic' family is even greater. Other allergic problems such as *asthma* and *hay fever* are also much less likely to develop in babies who are breast-fed. We now know that a whole range of disorders can be precipitated by allergy to cows' milk formula, including diarrhoea, vomiting, failure to thrive, bleeding from the intestine with subsequent anaemia, colic, nettle rash, a more or less permanent runny nose, a cough, wheezing and rattling of the chest and bronchiolitis.

The protection offered against allergy by breast milk is better understood by researchers nowadays and it is thought that just one feed of cows' milk formula can sensitize certain babies who later develop allergic symptoms. A very few breast-fed babies suffer from allergic problems while being breast-fed. One possible explanation for this is that foods which the mother has eaten (perhaps in excessive amounts) leak partly digested into the breast milk.

Breastfeeding a baby, especially exclusively, reduces the risk of his dying from a *cot-death*. There may also be some protection against the occurrance of *ulcerative colitis* and *Crohn's disease* in adulthood. Several fascinating studies have suggested that there may be a link between breastfeeding and protection against subsequent *degenerative heart disease*. Any conclusive answers will take years to work out but the hypotheses behind such suggestions seem so reasonable that there must at least be a glimmer of hope here for the prevention of angina and heart attacks. At present one in three middle-aged men in the Western world dies of heart disease so it's a ray of hope we can't afford to ignore.

It's a little-known fact that breast-fed babies are only half as likely to suffer from *dental decay* compared with bottle-fed babies; regardless of whether or not sugar is added to the cows' milk formula or whether the mother drinks water high in fluoride. Orthodontic specialists report that they see fewer problems with faulty *jaw and mouth development* in children who were breast-fed. This is thought to be because of the different sucking and swallowing actions seen in breast-fed babies.

There have been suggestions that breastfeeding may give some protection against the development of *multiple sclerosis* in adult life, though this is not proven. Other studies have suggested that children breast-fed for between four and nine months have relatively higher intelligence quotients, and that breast-fed children *walk* earlier.

As for the *psychological benefits* of breastfeeding to a baby, these are almost impossible to prove. However, one can reasonably assume that the baby breast-fed on an unrestricted basis and not left to cry but picked up and held for long periods may well grow up with greater feelings of security compared with a baby left to cry for long periods and given little physical comfort. The huge advantage of the breast to a baby is that it not only provides food and drink but also a source of comfort far greater than a bottle can ever offer.

The World Health Organization, the American Academy of Pediatrics, the Department of Health in the UK and many other health organizations have all agreed that breastfeeding is best for babies. There is no need to pretend otherwise. The final choice though, is of course up to each mother.

Reasons mothers give for and against breastfeeding

Reasons given by mothers of first babies for choosing to breastfeed (%)

Breastfeeding is best for the baby's health	83
Breastfeeding is natural	39
Convenience (no bottles to make up or sterilize)	38
Emotional satisfaction (closer relationship between mother and baby)	20
Influenced by friends or relatives	20
Influenced/advised by health personnel	18
Cheaper	17
Helps mother to get her figure back	8
Can't overfeed the baby	8
Don't know/no particular reason	3
Other reasons	4

Reasons given by mothers of first babies for choosing to bottle-feed (%)

Don't need privacy for bottle-feeding/would be embarrassed to breastfeed in front of others	43
Not tied to the baby because others can feed it	38
Don't like the idea of breastfeeding	25
Put off breastfeeding by experiences of others	17
You know how much milk the baby has had/don't need to worry whether he's had enough	14
Can't breastfeed for medical reasons/advised to bottle-feed by health professionals	9
Expecting to return to work soon	6
Don't know/no particular reason	5
Other reasons	7

(Percentages do not add up to 100 in either table as some mothers gave more than one reason.)

In our bottle-feeding society, it's inevitable that mothers will have strong feelings about how they are going to feed their babies. The large study of infant feeding in 1975 in England and Wales referred to earlier throws some interesting light on mothers' feelings.

What stands out very clearly from these two tables is that mothers choosing to breastfeed their babies are basing their choice on factors positively in favour of breastfeeding, whereas those deciding to bottle-feed give as their reasons factors *against* breastfeeding, *not* factors positively in favour of bottle-feeding. It's likely that the bottle-feeding mothers have simply never been exposed to successfully breastfeeding mothers who are enjoying the experience. It's also possible that they have never been told about the advantages of breastfeeding to their babies and to themselves. This information provides clear guidelines for those running ante-natal classes on how to discuss breastfeeding. Because mothers are influenced by information about the benefits of breastfeeding to the baby's health, these should be discussed openly, with no fear of making those subsequently choosing to bottle-feed feel guilty. All mothers deserve to be told the facts before making their decision and, given what we know, it would be irresponsible for health professionals to hide them.

The ante-natal period

Useful films for ante-natal classes include those giving mothers' views on breastfeeding. Having one or more breastfeeding mothers at the class for the other mothers to meet is also helpful, especially as even today some women have never seen a baby being breastfed. Discussion over such practical points as what clothes to wear so as to be able to breastfeed in public discreetly is useful, and the airing of feelings of probable future embarrassment at breastfeeding in front of other people − even close relatives − can help by enabling the women to realize that their worries are commonplace and can often be overcome with common sense and a sense of humour.

In all too many ante-natal classes breastfeeding is not discussed at all, though bottle-feeding is given plenty of time! Moreover, many mothers attending these classes don't come away with the impression that the person running the class is pro-breastfeeding, and this is unforgivable.

Society is at last slowly beginning to realize that boys and men need educating for parenthood just as much as women do. With today's small families of children born close together, neither boys nor girls get much practical experience of watching their parents rear younger children. The result is that the reality of having a baby in the house often comes as a shock to both men and women. People's attitudes and beliefs are formed slowly over the years and it is sensible to start discussing parenthood a long time before it becomes a fact. Some schools include classes on parenting, breastfeeding, family life and similar subjects in their syllabus, but it's essential that both boys and girls should discuss these matters openly. We live in a society with small, nuclear families often isolated from relatives and other support systems, and the understanding and support of the father are essential for the breastfeeding mother.

Ideally then, ante-natal preparation classes should put more emphasis on teaching couples. Discussions at such classes might include the benefits of breastfeeding to the baby and to the family; some common problems and whom to approach for help; and something about the sexual aspects of breastfeeding and the possible jealousy that can arise on the father's part. If parents-to-be have realistic expectations of what babies – and particularly breastfeeding babies – are really like, then they will be less surprised and more able to accept and cope when the time comes.

Most women need to buy bigger bras while they are pregnant and some of these are suitable for breastfeeding as well. The only requirements for a bra to wear while breastfeeding are that it should be quickly and easily openable and easy to do up, comfortable, not tight anywhere especially when the breasts are full, easily washed, and capable of giving the degree of support that a woman feels she wants. Ideally, it should also look attractive and not be built like a battleship. Many women find that while they are breastfeeding ordinary bras do just as well as special nursing bras. They are certainly easier to manage. If they are soft enough one of the cups can simply be pulled down to give the baby the breast, and there are no fiddly hooks and eyes to cope with.

One area in which women are given a lot of unnecessary advice during pregnancy is that of nipple preparation. Many women secrete colostrum from their nipples while they are pregnant, especially in the later months, but there is certainly no need to do anything more than to wash the breasts and nipples as usual. Rubbing or handling the nipples in an attempt to harden them has repeatedly been shown in surveys to make no difference to the eventual success of breastfeeding and probably puts a lot of women off. During the last few weeks of pregnancy it is good idea not to use soap on the nipples, as this makes the skin less able to stand up to the baby's sucking and more likely to become sore. There is certainly no need to use any creams, sprays or ointments on the nipples. Nature's own secretions take much better care of the skin than man-made equivalents can ever do.

If the nipples are actually inverted and don't stand out when the areola is held by a finger and thumb, it may be worth wearing plastic breast shells inside your bra to encourage the nipples to stand out. Many inverted nipples improve spontaneously during pregnancy even without this help.

The early days of breastfeeding

It's an interesting exercise to set the scene for the ideal environment in which the newly-delivered mother can start breastfeeding. She should feel at ease, whether she's at home in familiar surroundings or in a birthing room such as is used in some enlightened hospitals and birth centres. Conventional labour wards are not the most relaxing or comfortable places to be in but can be satisfactory if the staff are helpful and keen to encourage breastfeeding. She should also feel confident and relaxed with her birth attendants, who can share her feelings over the birth and in her first meeting with her baby. If she has been allowed to be upright during her labour, the odds are that she'll have needed few, if any, painkilling drugs, provided the labour was uncomplicated. She's also more likely to feel comfortable as episiotomies and tears are less likely in such an upright position.

The relaxed, comfortable, alert, upright (usually sitting at this time) mother can hold her new baby and has a chance to look at him, cuddle and examine him immediately after birth. The baby will fix his gaze on her eyes and have a good look around. He'll be attracted to her breasts by the look of them − the dark areolae are very noticeable − and by their smell. Pheromones produced by the skin have a distinctive smell and a newborn baby quickly learns to recognize his own mother's milk. At first he'll nuzzle and perhaps lick the nipple and areola. Next the so-called 'rooting reflex' will make itself evident. This is a searching movement for the nipple made when one side of the baby's mouth is stroked with the nipple. Finally, he'll take the nipple and part of the areola in his mouth and sooner or later will start sucking. It's important that he should be positioned well so that he can 'latch on' to the breast adequately and get the nipple well back into his mouth. What you don't want is for him to chew on the nipple alone and not to 'milk' the ducts beneath the areola properly. You can tell if he's swallowing if you see a small movement in front of his ears.

You'll probably feel some discomfort of your uterus as he sucks: this is caused by the contraction of the muscles of the uterus because of the oxytocin released into the bloodstream as the baby stimulates the nipple and areola. These contractions produce a sensation known as afterpains. After a while the placenta will come away.

Early contact like this has been shown in at least four major studies to make the mother more likely to breastfeed successfully and also to increase the length of time she's likely to continue breastfeeding. It also seems from research that there is a 'sensitive period' lasting around twelve hours after the birth. If mother and baby are separated during this period, subsequent breastfeeding may be affected adversely unless skilled support is available.

Virtually every painkilling drug that a mother is given during labour can get through the placenta into her baby and can make the baby sleepy and reluctant to suck in the first few days. Some drugs also cause jaundice which in turn makes the baby sleepy and disinterested in sucking. If you have too large a dose of such drugs, not only may you feel too doped to make the best of the first contact with your baby, but he may not demand as many feeds as he otherwise would until the fourth or fifth day.

Enlightened hospitals and midwives no longer separate a mother from her baby at all – even at night – from birth onwards. Success in breastfeeding is much more likely if there is absolutely no restriction of feeding patterns, either in their frequency of length, from birth onwards, and this is virtually only possible if the mother has completely open access to her baby *at all times*. Some hospitals now allow mothers to have their babies in bed with them and this obviously makes breastfeeding at night a much less laborious business as the mother then only has to get out of bed to change her baby's nappy. Studies show that mothers who keep their babies with them all the time are twice as likely to enjoy successful breastfeeding as are those whose babies are cared for in a hospital nursery.

Breast-fed babies rarely need anything but breast milk, provided their mothers are feeding them often and for long enough. If there is any restriction of sucking time or frequency, the milk will take longer to come in. Babies fed in an unrestricted way encourage the colostrum to become mature milk much more quickly and many such mothers experience their milk 'coming in' within twenty-four hours of the birth, instead of after two to four days, as happens if feeds are restricted. For the first day, colostrum − the first milk produced by the breasts − is quite adequate for the baby and indeed provides him with optimum amounts of nutrients and fluid, not to mention the invaluable anti-infective substances which babies given cows' milk formula or glucose water miss out on. The startling research finding that in England and Wales only 14 per cent of breast-fed babies were *not* given cows' milk formula puts our hospitals to shame, but in the last five years hospital practice has taken a turn for the better.

Most newborn babies like lots of feeds during the twenty-four hours. What's more, they do not drink all the time but enjoy simply holding the breast in their mouth and sucking every so often, perhaps as they drop off to sleep and find the nipple escaping from their mouth. This behaviour is quite natural and stems partly from the baby's inbuilt knowledge of how to stimulate the breasts to produce milk − that is, to hold and suck at the nipple and areola as much as possible; partly because each woman lets down her milk in an individual way, with the milk spurting out at intervals; and partly because each baby also has an individual sucking rhythm, with a pattern to the number of sucks and intervals between sucks per minute. What's more, some women don't let their milk down for several minutes after their baby has started sucking, so the baby may play at the nipple for that time, just sucking the 'foremilk' present in the ducts already until the 'hindmilk' from the milk glands is available.

When your milk comes in, you'll run the risk of becoming engorged unless you know how to prevent it. *Engorgement* simply means that the breasts are so full of milk that they are tense and tender. Pressure of the swollen milk glands tends to block blood vessels and lymphatics in the breast and fluid leaks out from these into the connective tissue. The skin over the breast is shiny and may be pitted like orange peel. It's liable to bruise and the breasts need handling gently. If you have engorgement, you'll feel hot and shivery and may sweat a lot. You'll also feel thirsty and there is no need to limit the amount you drink. Engorgement is more likely to occur in women who have been restricting the number and length of breast feeds, and so is usually seen on the third or fourth day after the birth. It may be no accident that this corresponds with the traditional time for women to suffer from the 'baby blues' — the day or so of weepiness often experienced. After all, engorgement is painful and causes a generalized bodily upset.

Engorgement is preventable simply by never letting the breasts become too full. Either put your baby to the breast to take off some milk, or *express* some if he really is too sleepy to feed. The midwife will show you how to express milk. Expressing nearly always takes much longer than putting the baby to the breast and letting him do the same job. It is an acquired knack and you'll need practice to get good at it. The milk won't be let down if you're anxious or embarrassed, so do it by yourself once you know what to do. Remember that to prevent engorgement you only have to take a little off. If you ever want to express enough milk for a feed for your baby, don't think your milk supply is inadequate because of the small amounts you get. Many successfully breastfeeding mothers never manage to express more than an ounce or two at a time, and have to collect milk throughout the day — perhaps after the baby has finished feeding each time — for one or more days in order to collect enough for one feed.

Sometimes your milk will flow enough to reduce the tension of your breasts if you sit in a hot bath. Ice packs or cold flannels can relieve the tenderness as well, as can aspirin. Your baby won't be able to latch on to your breast properly if it is engorged, so soften the areola first by expressing a little milk. If you have inverted nipples, you'll have to soften the breast and then perhaps use a breast shell inside your bra for a few minutes to bring the nipple out so your baby can take it properly. Obviously it is easier never to get engorged in the first place!

It's important to take care of your breasts while you are breastfeeding. Unfortunately, the very way in which we dress is likely to cause difficulties. Covering the nipples with absorbent pads of waterproof backed wadding, then putting on a fairly tightly fitting bra made of synthetic material, followed by layers of other clothing, many of them synthetic and so relatively non-absorbent, is not conducive to keeping the skin of the nipples in as good a state as possible to withstand the repeated episodes of sucking. The nipples sit there in a warm, damp, dark, airless atmosphere: just the right conditions for soreness to develop. If you use cream of any sort on your nipples, this increases the waterlogging effect, and soap is well known from many surveys to increase your chances of developing *sore nipples*. To prevent this, let some breast milk dry on your nipples after each feed, then keep your nipples dry, leave your bra off as much as you can and, if possible, expose your breasts to the light and air. Sunshine or an ultra-violet light can work wonders on really sore nipples. Make sure your baby is positioned well at the breast, is 'latched-on' properly and isn't putting undue suction on any one part of the nipple. Change his feeding position regularly to help avoid this. Finally, but most important, remember that research shows that you are actually *more* likely to suffer from nipple soreness if you restrict your baby's feed to the schedules so beloved by some old-fashioned maternity hospitals.

If you develop an actual *crack* of the nipple skin, you may find it is so painful that you have to use a rubber nipple shield for a day or two. Some women find that such a crack constantly re-opens. Try using different feeding positions in an attempt to take the pressure off that particular area of the nipple skin and let the light and air get to your nipples. If you find you have to stop feeding temporarily from the cracked side until it heals, express your milk regularly from the affected breast or use an electric breast pump. Your doctor may suggest an anti-infective cream as the crack can become infected with thrush or bacteria. The routine use of chlorhexidine spray does *not* prevent nipple soreness or cracking and is not advisable.

When you get your baby home you'll find breastfeeding easier in many respects. You'll be able to have the baby with you and in your bed if you want, and you won't be woken by other people's babies. However, you will have other things to do: the house to run, other children to look after, food to buy and prepare, and so on, and it's all too easy for breastfeeding to take second place. Once this happens, and once you start resenting the time you spend with the baby at your breast, you're well on the way to losing your milk. It's most important for breastfeeding mothers to relax enough to give their babies plenty of time. If you think this is easier said than done, try and get some help with running the house and family. Asking for help is nothing to be ashamed of and may be essential for the breastfeeding mother at home by herself for much of the day, especially if she has other children. Anthropologists put great importance on the *doula* figure who looks after, supports and encourages the breastfeeding mother in many communities all over the world. In our society the mother may feel that no one is playing this role. Her husband is probably out for much of the day and in any case has little understanding of the problems unless he is exceptional. Health professionals simply can't spare the time to fulfil the tasks of a *doula*, and lay breastfeeding counsellors are usually only available over the phone or for short periods during a visit. Today's mother, unless she is lucky enough to have helpful relatives living nearby, will have to rely on a combination of neighbours, friends, her husband, health professionals (a health visitor usually), lay breastfeeding counsellors and paid help to provide her with enough back-up for the important task she is undertaking. Their combined help should provide her with skilled advice on any problems that may crop up with breastfeeding; encouragement to carry out this advice; praise that she is doing well; company to keep her cheerful; and time to be with her baby. Instead of relegating the breastfeeding mother to another room to breastfeed, and making her feel embarrassed if she attempts to feed her baby in company, she needs to be helped to feel that she is doing a good job. Society's upgrading of motherhood starts here!

As for your *diet*, there is no evidence that any food or drink will increase your milk supply provided you are eating enough of a well-balanced diet. And fat stores you accumulated during pregnancy should slowly disappear, as long as you are not overeating. In countries in which women are malnourished, they still manage to feed their babies adequately at the breast for at least three months, though their own bodies may be depleted of calcium and protein, for example. If your normal non-pregnant weight is usually stable, then when you are breastfeeding you should eat slightly more than normal – about 300-500 calories a day extra, though this is only an average. You should drink whatever you want, though there is absolutely no need to drink a lot of – or indeed any – cows' milk. All the nutrients in cows' milk, though useful, can be obtained from other dietary sources.

Why mothers stop breastfeeding

We've seen that fewer than 1 per cent of mothers are still fully breastfeeding at four months after birth, even though the consensus of expert advice is that it is preferable to breastfeed for four to six months. Only 13 per cent are giving any breast milk at all at four months. Why is this? The same survey found some interesting, though not unexpected, answers.

Main reason given by mothers for stopping breastfeeding (%)

	Stopped by 6 weeks	Stopped between 6 weeks and 4 months	Stopped between 4 and 6 months
Insufficient milk	54	66	38
Painful breasts or nipples	12	4	6
Baby wouldn't suck/ rejected the breast	9	4	11
Inverted nipples	6	-	-
Mother ill	5	9	3
Baby ill	2	3	4
Had breast-fed long enough/ as long as planned	1	5	25
Breastfeeding too tiring/ taking too long	1	1	1
Domestic reasons	2	1	5
Embarrassment	2	1	-
Baby can't be fed by others	1	1	-
Didn't like breastfeeding	2	-	-
Going back to work	0	3	-
Other reasons	3	2	7
	100	100	100

Insufficient milk

Both these research findings and our own experience in dealing with mothers over many years show that the overwhelming majority of mothers stop breastfeeding before they had planned because they don't have enough milk to satisfy their baby. One criticism of this conclusion is that some mothers might secretly want an acceptable excuse to give people, when they actually want to stop for other reasons. However, the Department of Health survey was carried out by interviewers who were strangers to the mothers and who were never to be seen again, so there seems little reason for hiding their true reasons for stopping. Even if a few used 'insufficient milk' as an excuse, the proportion stopping for this reason is still extremely high.

Could it be that such a large number of women were actually *unable* to produce enough milk to nourish their infants? Simply from a common-sense standpoint the answer must be 'no'. There is no reason why two or three generations of bottle-feeding should have rendered the breasts of women in the West incapable of lactating. Natural selection and disuse take far far longer to effect genetic changes such as that and women had previously been successfully breastfeeding for five million years!

Another possible explanation suggested by some is that a particular environmental factor or behavioural characteristic makes Western women so unsuccessful at producing enough milk. The stresses of modern living and the lifestyle of young mothers may indeed make breastfeeding more difficult, but the fact is that vast numbers of women who have been unable to produce enough milk for their first, second or third children are able to breastfeed subsequent children quite satisfactorily when they are given the right advice and support. It is purely a problem of technique that stops women breastfeeding as long as they want: change the way they react to and feed their babies, and the breast milk is there. *All but a tiny proportion of women are perfectly capable of feeding their babies for as long as they want to, provided they know how to do it.*

This brings us back to the law of *supply and demand*. The more the baby is allowed to suck or play at the breast, the more milk will be produced. The phrase should really be 'demand and supply' because it is the baby's demands or sucking stimuli that create the supply, not the other way round. Maybe even 'demand' is a poor term, as it implies that the baby is being demanding and therefore something of a nuisance. Babies obviously have to make their desires to be fed known in order to survive and this can hardly be said to be a nuisance!

The trouble with much of the babycare information passed on to mothers this century is that it has largely been based on observations of bottle-fed babies. Bottle-fed babies tend to be happy on four-hourly feeds, partly because the relatively indigestible cows' milk formula stays in the stomach for about this time. All babies like to suck even when not getting milk, and whereas the bottle-fed baby will suck in air if allowed to suck on an empty bottle, and so has to be given a dummy or find his fingers for his 'comfort sucking', the breast-fed baby can enjoy the pleasant occupation of sucking at his mother's empty breast even when he's finished his milk. This has two important benefits. First the baby likes doing it, as you can see if you watch as he breaks off to smile and coo at his mother, then carries on sucking or playing with her breast. The interaction between a mother and her baby who is comfort sucking at her breast is quite different compared with that of a mother and baby who is sucking at a dummy. For one reason, the baby is necessarily being held by the mother and for another, she may well enjoy the feeling of her baby at the breast provided she is relaxed and has nothing pressing to get on with. The second important benefit is that the skin of the mother's nipple and areola are being stimulated by the baby even if he isn't actually sucking to get milk, and this has the effect of raising the level of milk-producing hormones just as sucking does when the milk is being let down. Many babies like to go to sleep while sucking at the breast. The only disadvantage of this to the mother is that she may feel she hasn't always got the time when the baby is ready for sleep.

Comfort sucking is much in evidence at night if the mother and baby sleep together, as they do in so many successfully breastfeeding peoples in non-Western communities. Compare this with our Western recommendations that babies should sleep in their own cots in their

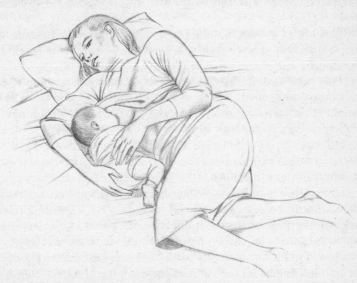

A restful way of feeding is to lie down. This is also the way some mothers feed their babies in bed at night.

own rooms. It's interesting that the advice of 'experts' on this matter doesn't in fact fit in with what parents do. Most parents don't banish babies to another room at night but keep them much closer, and increasing numbers are taking their babies into bed with them. The main problem seems to be simply one of small beds. Other 'dangers' such as crushing the child or his suffocating under the covers are almost non-existent, but if you are extremely obese, or take sleeping tablets, or if either you or your partner gets very drunk it is safer not to sleep with your baby.

The sort of breastfeeding practised in the West is really totally different in concept from that practised in many parts of the world and throughout history, quite apart from the fact that it is by and large unsuccessful. Instead of being simply a way of getting nourishment (albeit of the best kind) into babies, as is bottle-feeding, it should in fact be 'sold' to parents as an integral part of mothering and the mothering experience. One of the hormones produced during breast-feeding, prolactin, has been dubbed the 'mothering hormone', ('nature's tranquillizer') because it seems to promote feelings of relaxation and contentment in test situations in the laboratory. Quite apart from the pleasure the mother gets from the physical experience of the baby being at her breast, and the baby's obvious enjoyment, the effects of this hormone may put her in a different frame of mind from the bottle-feeding mother, whose prolactin levels quickly fall after childbirth.

Once breastfeeding is accepted as an integral part of mothering, a mother is more likely to put her baby to the breast at the least sign of unrest, rather than wait until the time has come for a feed. A breast feed becomes a time of mutual satisfaction as well as a way of comforting the baby and nourishing him. In some other countries breastfeeding is known as 'nursing' so as to get away from the idea that it is simply a way of feeding.

The mother who is feeding her baby at the breast in a natural, mothering sort of way will often find it difficult or impossible to say how many feeds her baby has had in a day. The frequency of feeds becomes unimportant to her, as does their length. Sometimes her baby will want to spend a long time at the breast – perhaps several hours on and off in the evening, especially in the early days – and sometimes he will want only a minute or two simply to get off to sleep. Contrast this with the mother feeding her baby according to the still-recommended schedules of six four-hourly feeds a day. If her baby is rash enough to cry between feed times he is highly unlikely to be offered the breast but may be jiggled about, given gripe water, a bottle feed or a drink of water, or simply left to cry until the right time comes for a feed of predetermined length. No wonder so many babies fed in this way suck so fast and furiously – they are 'clock-gobbling' in order to get their milk down in the short time they have learned is allowed to them at the breast.

The best way to get mothers to breastfeed successfully is never to recommend times or frequencies of feeds at all, but to 'allow' babies and mothers to get together as and when they want to. Sometimes a mother will need her baby to take some milk off, for instance if her breasts are tense and overfull, or if she has to go out shopping and wants to 'top the baby up' before they set off. Breastfeeding is a two-way affair, though usually the baby calls the tune. However, if you happen to have your baby in a hospital where schedules and routines are still advised, or if you yourself have chosen to breastfeed in a precise, mechanistic sort of way, you may find that you produce enough milk in spite of what has been said. Some mothers need relatively little stimulation to produce large amounts of milk, though to be fair they are few in number. If you are like this, your baby may well be satisfied, especially if his birthweight is above average. A few babies fall into a routine of their own which may sometimes correspond with a three-to five-hourly 'schedule'. Many mothers, however, will find that their babies will cry between feeds and won't put on enough weight if fed according to such a schedule. It is quite possible for a breast-fed baby to be apparently content and even to sleep through the night from an early age, and yet not be thriving and gaining enough weight. 'Happy to starve' is the term doctors have assigned to these babies, and their problem is quite simply that of insufficient milk.

To go back to the reasons given by mothers for stopping breastfeeding before they are ready, we can now see that the reason behind 'insufficient milk' is highly likely to be that they are doing what they assume to be right and so are feeding their babies too infrequently and for too short a time to stimulate their breasts to produce enough milk. It's surprising therefore that when the mothers giving 'insufficient milk' as their reason for stopping were asked what advice they had been given by their doctor, health visitor or midwife, 94 per cent replied that they had been told to give their babies complementary (top-up) bottle feeds of cows' milk formula or to stop breastfeeding completely and to put their babies on to the bottle! What they obviously should have been told to do at first was to put their babies to the breast more often (twice as often is a good guide), for longer times, ideally for as long as the baby wants to suck, and never to leave too long a gap between feeds. If a baby isn't demanding feeds by crying, then the breast should be offered, the baby being woken if necessary. The starving baby is often apathetic and sleepy rather than hungry and crying for the breast. A few of these babies might have needed more milk than the mother was ever capable of producing, but the vast majority of mothers would have been quite capable of *increasing their milk supply* to the levels needed by their babies.

In order to increase the milk supply, besides feeding the baby much more often and for longer periods (to increase the total amount of time the baby spends at the breast), it's important that the feeds should be spaced throughout the twenty-four hours. Long gaps of many hours at night, for instance, or even during the day if the baby has a long sleep can leave the breasts unstimulated for too long. The experience of breastfeeding mothers is that more milk is produced if there are never any really long gaps between feeds. It's quite possible to stimulate the milk supply by expressing or pumping milk, but the baby's sucking action is a much better stimulator of milk production than either of these methods, so it seems silly not to 'use' the baby. It appears that there is a latent period of about thirty-six to forty-eight hours before the milk supply increases after the number and lengths of feeds have been increased, and it is wise to be aware of this and not expect the baby to be satisfied as soon as you start giving more feeds. If your baby refuses to suck because there isn't enough milk there, you may have to express or pump milk temporarily until the supply increases two or three days later and he is satisfied again.

If you have been giving your baby complements of cows' milk formula and find he is reluctant to suck at the breast at all, you might like to try using a *Lact-Aid*, which is a piece of equipment designed to give the baby a stream of cows' milk formula through a fine polythene tube placed on the breast with its end on the nipple while he is sucking at the breast. In order to get the formula milk he has to suck hard, thereby stimulating the breast and increasing the supply of breast milk over a few days. Once the milk supply has been increased, the

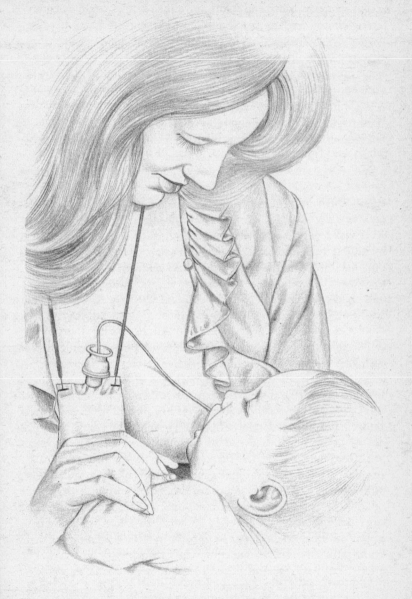

The use of a Lact-Aid

baby can usually be weaned off the Lact-Aid and cows' milk formula.

One of the problems behind the lack of knowledge about successful breastfeeding in our society as a whole, and among health professionals in particular, is that there is no one person or body of people who are expert on the subject. Many mothers and mothers-in-law either bottle-fed or breast-fed their babies on a tight schedule. Medical schools in general teach virtually nothing about the management of breastfeeding although matters are improving. Health visitor colleges have only recently begun to teach their students the principles of advising on how to breastfeed successfully, while there are so many schools of midwifery that the advice being handed out to student midwives has been a hotchpotch of the views of very large numbers of tutors, many in favour of bottle-feeding and most in favour of breastfeeding only if done according to schedules. The average breastfeeding mother has advice from about nine sorts of health professional including the ante-natal midwife, the labour ward midwife, the post-natal ward midwife, the community midwife, the health visitor, the general practitioner, the obstetrician, the paediatrician and the baby clinic doctor. Assume that each of these may be duplicated at least one because of shift work, weekends and holidays, and it is theoretically possible for a mother to be given a large amount of differing advice, depending on the individual views and education of each health professional. One American survey on the advice on breastfeeding handed out by paediatricians showed that they counselled mothers according to the experience their own wives had had of breastfeeding! One distinguished lecturer once told an assembled gathering of doctors that he never mentioned breastfeeding in lectures on infant feeding because it was too difficult! To get successful breastfeeding back on the map, not only do mothers have to be attuned to 'mothering through breastfeeding', but so also do health professionals and the rest of those in close contact with mothers. This can only be done by patient and well-informed health education on a large scale, and by local health authority decisions to co-ordinate advice on breastfeeding and to provide in-service training for their health personnel. In the long term, schools can do their bit as well, but the present generation of breastfeeding mothers needs help now — they can't wait for long-term remedies.

Returning to the table on page 71, the second most common reason for stopping before the mothers were ready in the first six weeks after the birth was *painful breasts or nipples*, though these were nowhere near as important as insufficient milk. Nipple soreness (see page 69); nipple cracks (see page 69); engorgement (see page 67); blocked ducts (see page 80); mastitis due to infection (see page 80); and breast abscesses (see page 81) are all more common in mothers breastfeeding in a restricted, scheduled way. Prevention is better than cure but if any of these conditions does occur the advice given needs to be based on a sound knowledge of the best way of overcoming the problem, and the mother will probably need lots of encouragement to carry on.

It's interesting that although *embarrassment* at the idea of breast-feeding prevents so many women from breastfeeding at all (see table, page 63), it is given as the reason for *stopping* by only 2 per cent of mothers who stop in the first six weeks. It's probably true to say, though, that many mothers might feel awkward at the thought of feeding on an unrestricted basis simply because it would necessarily involve feeding in front of other people sometimes, unless the mother were to go elsewhere every time her baby wanted to be at the breast, which would be a nuisance and likely to put her off the whole idea. Two factors are involved in this sort of embarrassment. One is that some babies make a lot of noise when they feed, sucking vigorously and making slurping noises. Other babies, especially when older, wriggle with pleasure when feeding, while others make a fuss and cry until the milk is let down. Few mothers in our society would be willing to carry on feeding this kind of baby comfortably in front of anyone other than people she knew very well. The other factor is that of nakedness. A lot of people imagine that in order to breastfeed a woman needs to bare her breasts. Nothing could be further from the truth. It is very easy to learn how to dress in order to breastfeed quite discreetly. Clothes that pull up from the waist such as jumpers and tee shirts are the most practical. Anything that unbuttons in front is likely to show much more naked flesh. It's true to say that if your baby is a quiet and calm feeder and if you are wearing suitable clothes, no one need know that you are doing anything other than cuddling your baby. It's interesting that women are said to feel most embarrassed at the idea of feeding their baby in front of their fathers-in-law. How much easier everything would be if society could stop being two-faced about breastfeeding and mothering. It's all very well for the experts to tell women that it's best if they breastfeed their babies, but unless society makes it easy for them to do so and stops making women feel awkward about doing it, they will continue to be put off unless they are very determined.

Some problems and situations you may experience

Blocked duct. If you find that an area of your breast is lumpy and tender, and the skin over it is red, you have probably got a blocked milk duct causing mastitis. It may be blocked because of the pressure from your bra or other clothing, from the way you were lying at night or because of general engorgement of your breasts as a result of letting too much milk build up in them. A blocked duct can recur because the baby always feeds in such a position that one duct in particular is never emptied properly. When you get a blocked duct you may have a raised temperature caused by substances from your milk being passed into your bloodstream. You may also feel 'flu-like and achey, weepy and bad-tempered.

First aid measures include checking that you have no clothing pressing on that area of your breast; emptying that particular area of the breast more frequently by letting the baby feed and then by expressing any residual milk; gently massaging over the lump towards the nipple after a feed; varying the position of the baby at your breast; varying the position in which you feed your baby; using hot or cold flannels, a covered hot water bottle or ice packs over the tender area to relieve the pain and to encourage drainage of the dammed-up milk; and taking aspirin if necessary.

As stagnant milk can become infected and cause infective mastitis or a breast abscess, it's wise to have a course of antibiotics if these first aid measures don't do the trick within twenty-four hours or so.

Mastitis (inflammation of the breast). The most common sort of infective mastitis, sporadic mastitis, follows an inadequately treated blocked duct. The area becomes more painful, hot and swollen and the skin looks shiny. Carry on the treatment for the blocked duct together with a course of suitable antibiotics from your doctor and try and get some rest. There is no need to stop breastfeeding, even temporarily, as the bacteria responsible are not harmful to the baby and are rarely present in the milk getting to the baby anyway.

'Epidemic mastitis' is seen earlier, often in maternity hospitals, and is caused by more virulent bacteria, often 'hospital staphylococci'. Several mothers may be affected at once. The bacteria originate from the baby's nose in many cases and may be traced back to a member of staff who is a carrier. The infection involves the milk ducts (unlike that in sporadic mastitis, which tends to involve milk which has leaked from the blocked duct into the tissues of the breast surrounding the ducts and glands). Sometimes pus can be squeezed from a nipple. The whole breast may be involved and the mother feels ill. Treatment with a long enough course of a suitable antibiotic (usually one of the newer penicillins) should be started following the despatch of a sample of milk to the laboratory for culture. While it is probably safe for the baby to carry on being fed at that breast, the safest course of action is to see what the bacterial count in the milk is. If it is high, the baby should be fed from the other breast and the milk supply in the affected side kept going by expression or pumping for a few days until the bacterial count has fallen. The breast should be emptied frequently and well to promote healing. Going home as soon as possible will remove you and your baby from the source of the original trouble.

Abscess. This usually follows inadequately treated mastitis. Provided an infected breast is emptied well and often enough and a sufficiently long course of an appropriate antibiotic is given, an abscess should be avoidable. Sometimes surgical drainage is necessary. To do this a surgeon makes an incision in the breast over the abscess. Once the pus drains, healing takes place within a few days. The milk from the affected breast should be discarded temporarily and the baby fed from the other side.

Blocked ducts and breast infections usually start in the first place because of poor feeding techniques with too few and too short feeds. Unrestricted breastfeeding is rarely associated with such problems.

Difficult feeders. There are many reasons why babies may not want to take the breast or may not feed well and there is no space here to go into all of them. Suffice it to say that whatever the reason (for example that the baby is affected by painkillers the mother had in labour; a poor feeding position is being used; the mother's nipples don't seem protractile; the breasts are engorged; the baby is tired because he has been crying and the hospital hasn't let you feed him;

the baby is full because he is still digesting a cows' milk formula feed given after your last breast feed; the baby was kept from you at birth; the baby is jaundiced; the baby has been given a bottle and likes the 'supernormal stimulus' of the large, easy bottle teat; the baby was smothered at the breast on one occasion; your milk takes several minutes to let down; the baby prefers one side; or the baby is over-whelmed by the gushing of your letting-down milk) *skilled help can nearly always put things right*.

Too much milk. This is most often a problem early on, when your newborn baby, particularly if he is fairly small, can be overwhelmed by the amount of milk being let down by your breasts. Sometimes the flow is so fast and furious that it is likened to a fire hydrant! If you watch the milk flow, you may notice that little jets shoot out quite haphazardly in all directions, and that one or more of these may be tickling his palate if he feeds in certain positions. Try keeping him off the breast until the initial flow has subsided somewhat. Try holding him in a different position – perhaps with his feet under your arm on the side you're feeding from. You could also try making him work harder for his milk: if you lie on your back, your milk flow won't have the force of gravity behind it.

Don't try to reduce your milk supply by feeding less often or for shorter times as your baby will soon need more and it is better if he adjusts your supply by his demands. Also, if you wait a long time between feeds, your breasts will be tense and full and the milk may flow even faster. You'll also lay yourself open to such problems as engorgement, a blocked duct or breast infection. If you are collecting a lot of milk that your baby doesn't need, give it to the local hospital milk bank.

The appearance of your milk. Breast milk varies in colour and consistency according to the stage of lactation and whether it is secreted early or late in a feed. Before your baby is born, you'll notice that your breasts produce small amounts of thin, bright yellow fluid which forms crusts on the nipples if allowed to dry. This is colostrum and continues to be produced, but in larger amounts, after birth. Colostrum contains very little fat and low levels of carbohydrates, but is rich in protein, certain minerals and vitamins, anti-infective sub-stances and live cells. It is extremely valuable to the newborn baby and very digestible and there is no reason to despise it just because it doesn't look like cows' milk and because there isn't much of it. It is better for your baby to have colostrum alone rather than to have feeds of cows' milk formula as well. Your colostrum will gradually change into mature breast milk – often within twenty-four hours if you are feeding frequently. At the beginning of the feed breast milk looks thin and sometimes bluish-white, whereas later on it becomes thicker and more cream-like in appearance. Sometimes the later milk is actually yellow. The difference in appearance is because of the different levels of fat: later in a feed more fat is present in the milk secreted by the milk glands. Never judge your milk by its appearance, provided you are producing enough. If you aren't producing enough, this is probably because your baby is spending too little time at your breast and your breasts are under-stimulated. In this case, your let-down may never get a chance to become established and you may produce only low-fat 'foremilk' for your baby.

Early on in a feed you may notice that some of the ducts opening at your nipple are secreting yellow milk while others are secreting whitish milk. This is quite normal and nothing to worry about. It simply means that some high-fat milk is already being let down or has remained there since the last feed.

As your baby weans, your milk will gradually decrease in amount and will become more like colostrum in appearance.

Premature babies. We've already seen how breast milk is slightly different in composition if your baby is born pre-term, and that this is very suitable for the needs of the baby. As for the ability of the baby to suck, a recent survey found that many babies are able to start sucking at the breast when they reach 1,300 g (just under 3 lb) and that by 1,600g (3½ lb) they can take all their milk at the breast. Before their sucking is this good, they still do best on breast milk, but it has to be given by spoon, or by tube passed down their nose to their stomach if they can't swallow. If the milk is given by bottle you run the risk of your baby always preferring the bottle to the breast. Keep your milk supply going by frequent expression or pumping and remember that four-hourly expressing or pumping is just as likely to lead to an inadequate milk supply as is four-hourly feeding of an older baby. You'll need a lot of skilled support and encouragement to carry on, but many women manage to breastfeed pre-term babies nowadays. Obviously it helps if there are facilities for you to sleep close to the nursery, and if your other children can be well cared for while you are in hospital with your baby.

Breast milk banks. Although a mother's own milk is better for her baby than is pooled milk from a milk bank, donated breast milk is still much better than cows' milk formula. Donor mothers are screened before their milk is accepted: their past medical history, blood tests and drug intake are all taken into account. As yet the best way of treating the milk in the bank is not agreed upon, but it seems that the less that is done to it within reason, the better, from the point of view of maintaining its anti-infective and immunological properties.

Caesarean section. After this operation you will find that it is difficult to get comfortable and you'll need to find ways of holding your baby that don't put pressure on your abdomen. An experienced nurse is invaluable at this time and you'll need someone there to pass you your baby and to hold him as you change sides. Feeding lying down with your baby next to you, and feeding in the 'twin' position with his legs under your arm on the side you're feeding from are two ways which may be comfortable for you. Experiment with pillows and don't worry about making a fuss over being sure you've found the best position. If you're uncomfortable, your let-down reflex is likely to be delayed or even to disappear completely.

   Other problems are that you may feel sleepy after your general anaesthetic, as may your baby. Calm perseverance together with frequent feeds by night and day should enable you to get off to a good start. If your baby is being nursed in a Special Care Baby Unit, try and arrange to be taken to him as soon as possible: there is no need to isolate yourself from him. Remember that your baby needs your breast milk just as much as if he were with you, and try to make sure that you get enough help to cope with expressing or pumping your milk if your baby is unable to suck.

Twins. Many mothers have breast-fed twins quite successfully and it's perfectly possible to make enough milk to nourish two babies: the increased demand simply stimulates more milk production. You'll save time if you feed both babies together, though if they are of different weights and different habits you may find that they usually

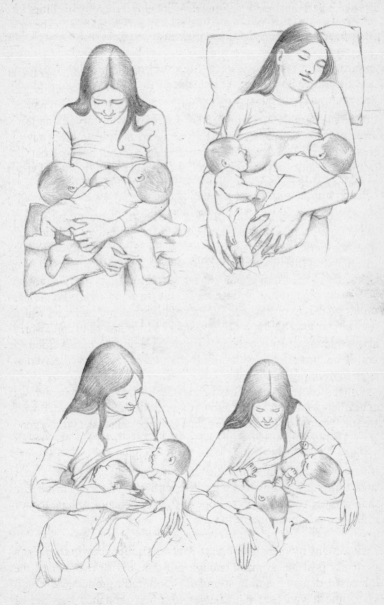

Several different positions for breastfeeding twins.

want feeds at different times. Experiment with feeding positions as there are several which make feeding two at once easier. Remember that your breasts make milk continuously, so there is no need to wait for any given time before putting one of the babies to the breast. Some mothers always put one baby to the same breast, while others have no such routine. Both methods are successful. At night you'll probably get more sleep if you feed your babies together or one after the other, waking one if you have to, rather than letting each wake spontaneously.

Adopted babies. Any woman can breastfeed a baby, her own or anyone else's, provided she builds up her milk supply by frequent and regular nipple stimulation. Having been pregnant, however long ago, makes it easier to do this, and the mother who decides to breastfeed an adopted baby will probably have to give her baby cows' milk formula complements if she has never been pregnant. A Lact-Aid (see page 76) makes building up the milk supply easier, as does plenty of skilled support and encouragement.

Relactation. Similarly, any mother can build up her milk supply to feed her baby again even if she stopped breastfeeding days, weeks, months or even years before. Again a Lact-Aid and skilled advice are helpful, together with lots of patience and perseverance.

Wet nursing. Wet nurses are no longer socially acceptable in the Western world today, though many babies might do better being breast-fed by other women while their mothers go out to work. However, some breastfeeding mothers feed each other's babies for the sake of convenience while one of them has to be away from her baby for a time. Giving milk to a milk bank is the modern form of wet nursing, though of course the baby misses out on being cuddled and sucking from the breast, albeit not his mother's.

Special situations. Certain disorders in the baby, for instance a cleft lip and palate, jaundice thought to be due to breast milk, or Down's syndrome, may call for skilled advice and management of breastfeeding. Don't be put off by people who advise you to stop breastfeeding simply because they haven't enough experience of helping mothers feed babies with these problems.

Certain illnesses in the mother, for example diabetes or tuberculosis, may similarly need particular knowledge to make sure that breastfeeding is safe for mother and baby. Very very rarely is it necessary for breastfeeding to be stopped in such women.

On the subject of the mother taking drugs of any sort and whether she should in that case breastfeed, the question to ask first is whether she really needs the drugs in the first place, because most drugs are secreted into breast milk and some have side effects in the baby. If a certain drug is essential and your doctor is not sure whether it is safe for your baby, there are several places where such information is available. There is a large and comprehensive list of drugs best avoided in our book *Breast is Best*. Research into drugs and breastfeeding is of necessity sparse, since it is not ethical to do trials of drugs in breastfeeding mothers unless they are warranted clinically. There are so few breastfeeding mothers actually taking any one drug that little may be known about the relative danger to, or side effects in the baby. Often the answer is to give the drug to the mother and to watch the baby for the appearance of any side effects, though certain drugs are known to be absolutely contra-indicated.

How long should breastfeeding go on?

There is really no answer to this as it is a matter for each individual mother and baby. However, an expert committee advising the Department of Health and Social Security in the UK recommended that all babies should be breast-fed for a minimum of two weeks and preferably for four to six months. Unfortunately the wording was not very detailed, probably because they didn't feel they could make specific recommendations at that time (1974), and the word 'fully' (breast-fed) was left out. However, from the point of view of avoidance of allergy and infection alone, it is full breastfeeding (that is, with no other food or drink given to the baby which confers maximum protection in the first four to six months. Similarly, the wording implied that after four to six months it didn't matter what happened. There is some evidence to suggest, though, that from the point of view of the baby's physical health, there are some advantages to breastfeeding continuing beyond this time, and certainly we just don't know enough about the baby's emotional and developmental aspects to suggest that breastfeeding should be discontinued at this time. Patterns around the world today and throughout history have been that breastfeeding continues for several years until the next baby comes along. Even four to six months seems puny by comparison with this ideal situation. (For a discussion of this see page 13.)

In parts of the world where successful breastfeeding is still the norm and where Western ideas have not yet infiltrated and spoiled things, babies are breast-fed for several years. Other foods are given as well from the latter part of the baby's first six months of life, and of course breast milk assumes a less and less important role nutritionally as the baby grows older and takes in more calories in the form of other foods and drinks. The baby has the advantage, though, not only of the pleasure of the close relationship with his mother while he is still allowed to go to the breast, but also of a supply of easily digestible food if he is ill. He can also be readily comforted at the breast, though he spends less and less time there as he grows older.

In areas where there is insufficient food available, and where illness due to malnutrition is rife, a young child's lifeline may be his supply of breast milk. When he is finally taken off the breast, for instance when the next baby is born, he runs a risk of potentially fatal diarrhoea and malnutrition. As long as the new baby is given priority, there is, of course, no need to take the older child off the breast and it is often safer in such circumstances not to do so. In areas such as these, any extra food supplies should be channelled to the breastfeeding mother rather than only into weaning foods for her baby. In the Western world, a mother who is already breastfeeding may be under social pressure to stop doing so if she becomes pregnant again, but there is no other reason why she should.

Contraception

Worldwide, breastfeeding is still the most important contraceptive. Where completely unrestricted breastfeeding by day and night is the norm, and where the breasts are never left unstimulated for more than a short time, babies are spaced at two to three-year intervals solely by breastfeeding contraception. Breastfeeding delays the return of ovulation after childbirth in such women. Because ovulation can occur before the first period after childbirth (though the first cycle or so is commonly anovular), breastfeeding contraception is obviously not popular in countries requiring totally reliable

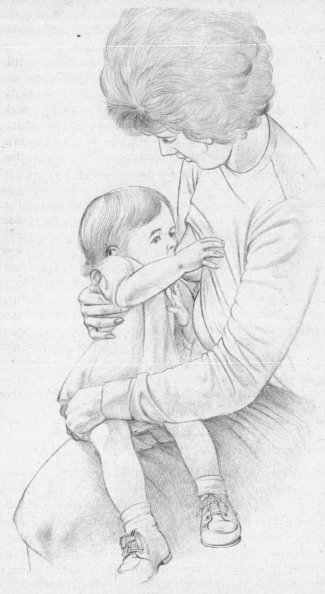

Breastfeeding an older child.

contraceptive techniques. However, given that it has been estimated that in the USA among women feeding their babies at the breast in an unrestricted way ovulation takes an average of fourteen months to return, many couples may consider breastfeeding to be a very suitable method of spacing babies, especially as it has no side effects. From research in the USA it seems that the use of a dummy (which prevents a baby from sucking at the breast in an unrestricted way), the baby sleeping for long periods (such as at night), and the giving of food or drinks other than breast milk can all speed up the return of ovulation.

By giving up breastfeeding, the Western world's women have given up an integral part of their function as women. They have also put their children at risk, though this risk is reduced with modern health care. They may have put themselves at a greater risk of suffering from certain disorders. They have also discarded without thinking not only a convenient way of feeding their babies and a way of spacing their family, but something that leads, inevitably, to a close and warm relationship with their children. Women who choose to breastfeed in an unrestricted way are unanimous that this method beats bottle-feeding and 'token' breastfeeding every time.

CHAPTER 4

Breasts and sex

As we saw in Chapter 1 the function of the female breast is twofold — sexual attraction and the feeding of infants. We have looked at breast-feeding in Chapter 3 and in this chapter we'll look at the breasts as sex organs.

Human beings are exceptional in the animal world in that breasts develop before they are needed to suckle the young. We don't know why this happens but we can only assume that the breasts of the human female are there beforehand to act as an erotic stimulus to encourage mating. And this they certainly seem to do, albeit in varying degrees across the different cultures of the world. Having said this, though, it is probably mainly in the Western world, and in America in particular, that the breasts have become *the* erotic focus.

Today's women are probably more obsessed with their breasts than ever before, partly — if not entirely — because today's men are similarly obsessed. As we said in Chapter 1, in a world in which women often have short hair and wear trousers, do men's jobs and are generally eroding men's traditional roles, men (and to a lesser extent women themselves) see breasts as the one sexual difference they can't hide or negate and so if anything emphasize them. The media and the girlie magazines in particular worship breasts in a totally unnatural way which makes women feel insecure and men dissatisfied. Clever photography and posing can do wonders for a modestly endowed woman but the average woman doesn't know this and wonders why she too can't look like the pneumatic beauties her partner so admires. This leads her to buy more uplifting bras and, increasingly today, to cosmetic surgery.

Our society's admiration for the big-breasted woman stems in part from the Hollywood era of film stars with hourglass-shaped figures. Since the 1940s boys have grown up with the idea that big breasts are sexy. Not only are big-breasted women thought to be intrinsically more interested in sex, but their very appearance is traditionally thought to carry more sex appeal to men. The combination of looks plus the fact that the men believe such women are more interested in

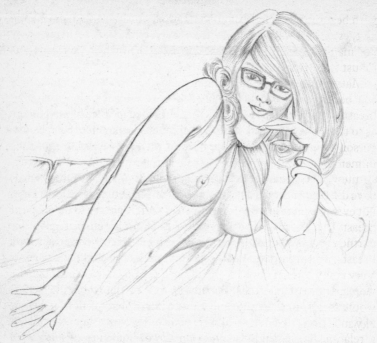

A classical 'boob' shot from a men's magazine of the '60s. An example of how the media pander to some men's concept of the ideal breast.

sex conspire to make men (especially those over forty-five or so) very attracted to big breasts.

It may be true to say that *some* women who grow up with relatively big breasts are more interested in sex than their smaller-breasted sisters. From adolescence onwards they will have been unable to ignore the interest their shape arouses in men and, indeed, in other women, and they cannot help but be aware that big breasts are considered sexy. The woman who is relatively uninhibited and finds men attractive may well be more obviously interested in sex. Not only does she have more chance to get to know men because of their interest in her but she is aware of their admiration for her breasts.

The danger for big-breasted women comes when they start believing that their sex appeal starts and ends with their breasts. It is a very superficial relationship which is based only on each partner's tacit awareness of the beauty of a part of one of their bodies! Women with beautiful faces have often found themselves in a similar situation and, even worse, have found — like several film stars — that not only one man but society generally believes that their whole value amounts to just a pretty face.

Mature men and women understand that small-breasted women can be just as sexy and can have just as much sex appeal as big-breasted women. This is not to say though that individual preferences as to the looks of breasts shouldn't exist. It's impossible to wipe out a person's culturally inherited values of physical beauty. From time immemorial different peoples have had their own ideas of what constitutes ideal female physical beauty, and many of these ideals have differed enormously from those of our society today. In any case, not everyone agrees with currently held preferences as to the shape of breasts, which is a good thing! If every man were satisfied only if his partner had big breasts, half of all women (the 49 per cent whose breasts are by definition below average in size) would feel spurned. Very many couples have a happy, loving relationship even though the woman's breasts are not what the man — or the woman herself — would ideally like. Few people achieve physical perfection (if there is any such thing) in any area of their bodies. The success or otherwise of a relationship depends far more on the personalities of the couple involved than on what they look like, and this is how it should be.

Interestingly enough, it seems that society's ideal breast image is slowly changing anyway. The ideal woman as portrayed by the media is neither very slim nor very curvy. She is neither particularly big nor small-breasted. This perhaps reflects the enormous variety of fashion, hairstyles, make-up, popular music and drama available today, which are incomparable with the concept of a stereotyped woman. Women are at last expecting to be appreciated for their worth as people and this expectation is being increasingly recognized. No longer does a woman have to have a certain 'look' for people to find her attractive. They are far more likely to look at whether a woman takes care of her body and makes the best of herself, at how interested in everything she is, what her beliefs and views are and, of course, at what sort of personality she has. Some of today's most successful film stars and pop idols have small breasts. It would be interesting to see if it were possible to age a man by his views on the ideal breast! It seems likely that men preferring bigger breasts would on average be older, having been influenced by a different generation's ideals.

Because of society's natural enjoyment of the breast as a sexual organ we're wide open to its exploitation in an age of 'sex is for pleasure' and two babies (at most) per couple. For most couples the main function of the woman's breasts is sexual simply because she breastfeeds either very little or not at all. This makes us very vulnerable to the advertising world and to the commercial exploitation of breasts generally.

All of this has a potent and lasting effect on a young girl as she grows up. Girls compare their breast development with each others' and with their mothers' both in reality and in fantasy and for most girls their breasts are the first manifestation of their awakening sexuality. They are intensely proud of them. At first this produces an ambivalent attitude and a sense of guilt as men (and particularly their fathers) begin to notice that they aren't little girls any more but young women. Many young girls hide their breasts from their fathers as they are budding. They do this for two reasons. First, about this time many girls are going through an Oedipal stage in which their fathers becomes attractive to them as males and second, they feel (quite subconsciously) that by flaunting their breasts they may be seen to be competing with their mother in their father's eyes. Many adolescent girls, when asked, say that their breasts are much nicer than their mother's and that theirs will never droop or become unattractive. Indeed, their firm young pointed breasts probably *are* more aesthetically pleasing than those of their mother's generation. At this stage many girls are so confused and guilty about their awakening sexuality that they hide their breasts from the outside world by wearing tight clothes and by putting off buying a bra that accentuates their breasts at all.

As the young girl advances in her teenage years, though, she begins to realize that her breasts give other people (and her) a lot of pleasure. Psychologists and analysts have had a field day trying to explain why teenage girls feel the way they do about their breasts and opinions vary enormously. Freudian analysts, for example, maintain that girls see their developing breasts as a consolation prize for not having been given a penis and that a girl's first dealings with her breasts are all homosexual (among girl-friends) as opposed to heterosexual. This penis envy story has, deservedly in our opinion, come under a lot of fire and most analysts now have a more balanced view of the subject.

As a young girl's breasts develop she experiments with handling them and soon finds that it feels good. Some girls go through a phase of allowing other girls to play with their breasts and this is completely normal. All of us go through a homosexual stage during our sexual development but this is usually a prelude to hetrosexual relationships. Once heterosexual contact starts a girl realizes that boys like her breasts and so makes the most of it. At this stage the breasts become important sexual symbols and she starts to buy bras and to wear clothes that accentuate what nature has given her.

Fashions, advertising and male conditioning all contrive to make women increasingly breast-conscious and although many women do not see their breasts as being of especial sexual significance compared with the rest of their bodies, they are virtually forced to do so by pressure from outside. This leads many women to see the role of their breasts as exclusively sexual. In fact, most women never consider any other role for them. This means that when anything goes wrong (they find a lump, for example) they are terrified to go to a doctor just in case it means that their main sexual symbol will have to be removed. As we shall see, the average woman with a lump waits for six months before seeking medical help. This simply wouldn't occur if the lump were on her foot or another less sexually important part of her anatomy. Not only does this over-emphasis on the sexual nature of the breast mean that many women die needlessly because they can't bear to go to a doctor with their lump, but it also means that millions of babies never have the best start in life that they deserve – breastfeeding. There is a whole chapter on this vital function of the breasts but here we shall look a little more at the sexual implications of breastfeeding.

Breastfeeding is for many woman a deeply satisfying and even sexually pleasant experience, as in historical terms it has had to be: if it hadn't been women wouldn't have fed their children who would therefore have died. But to link breastfeeding (a reasonable *nutritional* practice in the eyes of many women) to sexual feelings is too much for most women. If they experience anything other than a mildly 'pleasant' sensation they feel guilty and may even give up breastfeeding altogether. Many women have told us that they felt bad about feelings of sexual arousal while breastfeeding and some have even said that when experiencing these feelings when feeding a boy they felt disgusted because it was 'so incestuous'. Yet nearly two-thirds of all the women in our survey who had breast-fed said that they had found the experience 'sensual' or 'sexually pleasant'.

Unfortunately society has become so hung up on intercourse as the only form of sexual expression that many people ignore or deny the richness and variety of sexual feelings that are available. Women especially are plentifully endowed with several different ways of obtaining sexual pleasure, all of which are inextricably interlinked. Men by comparison have a very poor repertoire, concentrating as they do on intercourse as their main source of sexual enjoyment.

Sexual arousal and the female breast

During the earliest phase of sexual arousal the first sign that anything is happening is that the nipples become erect. This comes about as the tiny smooth muscles in them contract. One nipple often erects before the other and erection can occur even without physical stimulation. Stimulation either by the woman herself or by her partner usually hastens erection but is not essential. The nipples increase in length and diameter as the woman becomes more excited and blood collects in and around them. This mechanism is rather like that which causes a penis to become erect.

The size of the breasts and nipples has no bearing whatsoever on how responsive they are sexually. Some women have exquisitely sensitive nipples which, when stimulated, bring them to orgasm within seconds whilst other women are almost totally unresponsive. Nipple length during sexual arousal may increase by up to 1 cm (½ inch) and nipple width by ½ cm (¼ inch). Average-sized nipples increase in size proportionately more than do larger ones. By and large mouth stimulation (sucking and gentle licking) produces faster nipple erection than does stimulation with the fingers but obviously this varies from woman to woman.

Once the nipples are erect the patterns of veins on the breasts often become more marked and the breasts begin to swell – sometimes by as much as 30 per cent of their usual volume. This swelling is most obvious in women who haven't breast-fed. Later on in this *excitement phase* the areolae swell and the breasts may become covered with a faint red flush or measles-like rash which can also cover the abdomen and neck. Some women don't have a sex flush at all and in others it appears very late. About three-quarters of women, though, do have a sex flush like this just before orgasm.

The next stage of sexual arousal is known as the *plateau phase*.

During this the breasts swell more and the areolae especially become swollen. This swelling may be so marked that it makes the nipples appear shorter. In fact the nipples are usually still swelling at this stage but are masked by the swelling of the areolae.

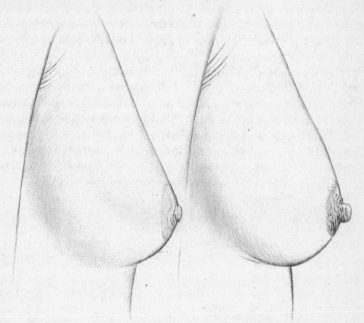

The same breast before (*left*) and during (*right*) orgasm.

At *orgasm* itself women experience all kinds of sensations of which some are related to their breasts. Some women like their breasts or nipples held very hard or even squeezed as they have an orgasm but because the intensity of the other changes in the body is so great it is easy for a man to hurt his partner's breasts or nipples as she 'comes off' because she is much less sensitive to pain for these few brief moments. It makes sense to draw a line between what a couple finds pleasant and stimulating and what seems to produce damage. This is particularly true of biting the breasts or nipples during intercourse. Bites can produce infections so care is called for.

It's probably fair to say that with the exception of the very 'breast-erotic' woman, caressing the breasts is much more stimulating to the man than to his partner. This means that a woman to whom breast stimulation is unimportant may well only enjoy her breasts sexually as a way of exciting her man. This is perfectly acceptable – after all, making love is a selfless pursuit in which both partners seek to give pleasure as well as to receive it.

Once orgasm is over about the first thing to happen is that the areolae return to normal. This marks the onset of the final phase of the sexual arousal cycle – *the resolution phase*. This change in the areolae gives the impression that the nipples are becoming erect again but it isn't so. They are simply more visible as the surrounding areas subside. This increased prominence of the nipples is a good sign that a woman has has an orgasm. The sex flush fades and the breasts return to their former unexcited size. At this stage many women don't want their breasts touched because they are exquisitely tender or so pleasantly 'satisfied' that further stimulation is positively unpleasant. Unlike men, though, many women are capable of several orgasms in succession and soon the breast is ready for a new excitation phase.

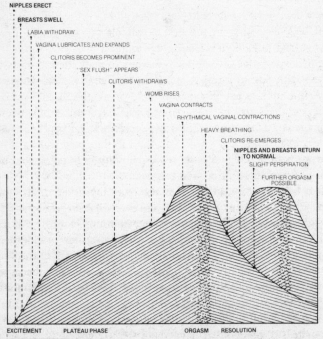

The sequential changes that occur in a woman during sexual arousal.

This sexual arousal cycle occurs every time a woman has an orgasm whether by masturbation or with a lover. Lesbians always say that they understand what women want much better than men do, and put great stress on sensitive and prolonged breast play. About half of all women say they like their breasts to play a part in their lovemaking but our research and that of others suggests that this may be an underestimate because so many women feel so guilty about sex or so ill at ease with their breasts they won't let them be used sexually. One of the saddest findings of our research was that men were not doing to women's breasts what women most liked to be done. That vast majority of women generally complain that men are too rough (especially squeezing their breasts too much); put too much emphasis on breast play too early in sexual arousal; are too selfish about what they do and rarely ask what the woman herself wants. Many women (38 per cent in our series) admitted to playing with their breasts or nipples when they masturbate (and probably more than this actually do so) and so can easily tell a man what they most like, if only he would ask. It's up to a woman to tell her lover what she likes and to school him in doing it until he pleases her in the best possible way. Lovemaking isn't a self-centred behaviour: it is by definition a two-way, mutually enjoyable experience. By and large women want their breasts to be played with late in foreplay and then very gently and lovingly. The only time most women want any kind of roughness (if indeed they want it at all) is very late on around orgasm. A number of women find their breasts are so sensitive during pregnancy, late in the menstrual cycle and in some cases while on the Pill that they can hardly bear them to be touched at all, yet some men persist in doing so much to their partner's discomfort and annoyance.

The lactating breast is just as erotic as any other. Many women spurt milk as they have an orgasm and even mild sexual arousal causes leaking in others. There is absolutely nothing wrong with a man sucking his partner's nipples when she's lactating – indeed many couples get a lot of pleasure from doing just this once they know it isn't perverted in some way. So many couples think that because the woman is feeding a baby her breasts must cease to be sexy to the man. This is crazy and is just another reason so many men are anti-breast-feeding. After all, if you've always seen your partner's breasts as your favourite sex objects, to have them denied you is very bad news indeed. But they don't have to be. There is absolutely no reason why as the baby sucks one side the man can't suck the other if he wants to. A breast-centred woman will like it. Many couples have the sexiest time of their lives during breastfeeding because the woman is very breast-centred and is not having to bother with contraception because she's not ovulating (see page 88). Many women feel permanently slightly aroused when they're breastfeeding and this has dividends for their partners.

This is all part of a perfectly well-documented and natural series of events. Successful procreation depends on three pleasant phenomena in women: intercourse, childbirth and breastfeeding. These are closely related physiologically and psychologically and many a psychosexual counsellor knows that the same qualities that make a good lover also make a good mother. A woman who relates to her body easily and enjoys pleasurable intercourse with ready orgasm is more likely to enjoy pregnancy, giving birth and breastfeeding her baby. It is all part of the continuum of her sexuality.

Many observers have noted that the reactions of a woman's body during orgasm are noticeably parallel to those when she is giving birth. Many obstetricians have noticed that the clitoris often enlarges during childbirth and that this is especially likely to occur if the husband is in the room. Masters and Johnson reported on twelve women in labour who described it as being as intensely pleasurable as an orgasm.

During breastfeeding, too, many women become sexually aroused, albeit usually not to orgasm. During an orgasm the uterus contracts, the nipples erect and the breasts swell. Exactly similar changes occur during breastfeeding and indeed during childbirth. Women who breastfeed have been shown to be more tolerant in other sexual areas, to be generally more sexually 'together' and to return to intercourse after childbirth earlier than their non-breastfeeding sisters.

So clearly breasts can be a wonderful source of pleasure to a woman at many different stages of her life and the sexually at ease woman makes the most of it. Even after the menopause most women still find their breasts sexually arousing so there's no reason to believe that the end of one's reproductive life marks the end of one's breasts as erotic centres. It's very difficult to chart breast awareness and how it arises but there is no doubt that some women are very much more breast-orientated than others. Women who are very aware of their breasts are more likely to have multiple orgasms and a woman who enjoys her breasts will continue to do so long after their potential for biological function is over.

Breastfeeding, orgasms and childbirth share common biological mechanisms and are all based on three basic female characteristics. First, they all involve the same complex and interlinked hormonal and neurological pathways; second, they are very sensitive to environmental stimuli and are easily inhibited in their early stages; and third, they seem to be a prelude to 'caring' behaviour. There has been a fair amount of animal research to back this up. Three Belgian researchers, for example, joined the circulatory systems of pairs of sheep, using plastic tubes to connect their jugular veins. In some pairs they joined rams with breastfeeding ewes and massaged their penises and testicles to orgasm. Within thirty seconds there was a sharp rise in pressure in the ewes' udders. Their milk ejection reflexes had been stimulated by the blood of the sexually stimulated rams.

In other research two ewes were joined by their blood circulations and the vagina of one distended with a balloon to simulate what happens during intercourse and breastfeeding. Stimulation of one ewe's vagina produced milk ejection in the other.

But very little comparable work has been done in humans and even today in the 'permissive' 1980s there is much we still don't know about the breast as a sex organ. A lot more research could be done.

Women are exceptionally sensitive about the appearance of their breasts in a sexual setting. Women with small or asymmetrical breasts feel they'll be at a disadvantage, as do women with inverted nipples. Those with large, pendulous breasts fear they'll put men off and those with scars after surgery are even more upset. A woman who has had her breast removed by mastectomy has special, and understandable, problems which are considered in more detail on page 192.

We cannot stress too strongly that a woman's intrinsic enjoyment of her breasts has nothing whatsoever to do with their anatomical appearance. If ever a problem was 'all in the mind' this one certainly is. Unfortunately, because of a repressive upbringing and hosts of other reasons, many women enter adulthood with a very poor body image, especially of their breasts. They then become brain-washed by pin-ups, advertising and the media generally and by some men's totally unrealistic expectations into believing that only perfectly shaped and contoured breasts will attract a man. This is one of the most dangerous and destructive myths of our day and leads countless millions of women to experiment with ways of enlarging their breasts, most of which are useless, except cosmetic surgery which has its hazards and is very expensive. There is probably very little that can be done about this ridiculous state of affairs in a breast-orientated society except perhaps to change people's attitudes towards breasts over many years and to start looking at women as whole human beings. That this attitude is deeply offensive to women generally (and not just to 'women's libbers') is perfectly understandable.

Hopefully, today's aware parents will start their daughters off on the right road by behaving in a balanced way to their breast development. Fathers (or indeed any other member of the family) should never tease their budding daughters because it can be too much for their sensitive sexual psyches to accept at that age. The damage done by a father's thoughtlessness or hurtful remarks can remain with a girl for life. Unfortunately her partner often ends up reaping the harvest of this seed – not her father. Breasts should never be made to seem 'dirty' or 'wrong' to a young girl – or indeed to anybody. If a young girl were not to become aware of her breasts as being sexual she would be abnormal. If a girl is made to feel sinful or wrong for allowing a boy to touch her breasts she'll carry that guilt with her for years and possibly even for ever. Children should never be led to believe that breast play could lead to cancer. There is absolutely no truth in this. There is no evidence at all that any form of sexual activity (including practices in which the breasts come into contact with the penis or semen) causes cancer or any other diseases. A woman who is destined to get some kind of breast condition will get it anyway whatever her sexual practices. In fact there is some evidence that intercourse without the use of barrier methods (that is methods that allow semen to bathe the woman's cervix and vagina) might even have a protective function against breast cancer. For more details of this see page 171. Similarly there's no evidence that powder, perfume or anything else used on the breasts does them any harm. Perfume should be kept off the nipples because it's not pleasant for the man to taste but that's the only reason. Nipple stimulation may become unpleasant because of tenderness around the time of the menopause but a loving couple will find ways to overcome this problem. Anyway, nipple and breast play have no effect on the progress of the menopause and can, of course, be continued after it.

Finally, be careful how you use your breasts sexually. Don't dress in a way that accentuates them, wear jewellery to draw attention to them, or rub them against a man and then wonder why he makes a grab for them unless you are happy and able to cope with the consequences. Breasts are a very powerful sex symbol for most men and if they are flaunted can easily bring them more attention than you really want.

It's up to each of us to help put breasts back where they belong in the perspective of human sexuality, just as one attractive part of a whole person.

CHAPTER 5

Some common problems

One in four women in the Western world will have some kind of breast condition during her lifetime. Of these the vast majority are harmless and some simply a nuisance. In this chapter we look at the commonest problems women have with their breasts, leaving the subject of cancer (apart from passing references) until Chapter 8.

Hair on the breast

The breasts, like the rest of the body, are covered with hair, the distribution and amount of which is inherited. Some women are generally more hairy than others and their breasts are no exception.

In our culture it is not usually considered sexually attractive to have excess body hair and many men find hair on and around the breasts a sexual 'turn-off'. Hair around the areola is not at all uncommon and is more noticeable in women with darker complexions.

Excess hair that bothers either partner can be shaved, plucked, removed with depilatory creams, or removed permanently by electrolysis. Most women pluck out the obvious hairs and leave less obtrusive ones but there is no doubt that electrolysis is the only permanent answer to the problem. In this procedure a beautician uses an electrode that delivers a tiny electric current to the root of the hair. It is a very time-consuming procedure because each hair follicle has to be treated individually, but as the growth of hair around the nipple is usually not very lush this isn't quite such a problem as it is elsewhere on the body. If it is too painful it can be done under a local anaesthetic. How many visits you'll need to make depends on how much needs to be removed. When done by a properly qualified operator the hairs will not grow back because the hair-producing follicles have been killed. Removing hair by electrolysis is a relatively skilful business. As the hair follicles may not be straight and are usually at an angle to the skin surface, one dose of electrolysis may not kill the root of the hair and each follicle may need to be treated several times.

There is no evidence that removing chest or breast hair by any other method makes it grow back thicker or more vigorously and undoubtedly the vast majority of women use simple home methods rather than expensive and time-consuming electrolysis. Bleaching the hair is another inexpensive way of camouflaging the problem.

Hormones produced by tumours of the ovary and adrenal glands can produce excessive hair growth but the Pill and hormonal changes of pregnancy do not. If you notice a sudden growth of hair all over your body, see your doctor.

Breast pain (mastalgia)

Breast pain is a sensation that most women have experienced. Many have it regularly before every period while others just get the odd bout from time to time. Unless it is a regular monthly occurrence it's easy to worry that the cause might be a cancer. Cancer is, however, not a common cause of pain in the breast.

In many hospitals around the world there are now breast pain clinics and in recent years the subject of breast pain has been studied more closely than ever before. These studies have categorically refuted the long-held (male) medical view that pain in the breast was a psychoneurotic condition. Breast pain is now recognized as having various causes the *least* important of which is neurosis. Because doctors accepted the findings of various studies in the 1930s and 1940s which suggested a psychological basis for breast pain, little was ever done to help women with this very real problem. This has all changed in the last decade and breast pain is, rightly, treated as seriously as pain anywhere else.

The reason that this change in attitude has come about is that modern investigative methods such as thermography, mammography, xeroradiography, hormone measurements and better pathological techniques have been brought to bear on the problem. Surveys have shown unequivocally that women with breast pain are no more neurotic than those without it and the symptom has at last become 'respectable'.

Women of all ages may suffer from breast pain but it seems to be most common between the ages of thirty and fifty. The sensations usually described are 'heavy, as if full of milk', 'sharp', 'cutting', 'burning', 'drawing', 'gathering', 'aching', 'bruised', 'stabbing' and 'sore'. No specific descriptive term is used by women who have a cancer as their cause of pain. Approximately twice as many women have pain in the left breast compared with the right and about one in eight have pain in both breasts at the same time. Two-thirds of the women studied in one piece of research complained that the pain radiated outside the breast itself – often to the armpit or arm. Some women's pain is worst at night and some lose sleep because of it.

Let's look now at each of the main causes of breast pain in turn. We won't consider pain-producing lumps in the breast because treating such lumps usually cures the pain and lumps are discussed elsewhere (see page 115).

By far the commonest cause of breast pain is a condition known as *cyclical pronounced mastalgia* (cyclical mastalgia or mastalgia). In this syndrome the pain only occurs, or is worse, during the pre-menstrual days and is a manifestation of fibrocystic disease (see page 119). It is distinguished from the normal physiological pain that many women have pre-menstrually by the fact that it is 'pronounced', more intense or more persistent, sometimes lasting for up to three-quarters of the menstrual cycle. The pain is difficult to localize but if it is anywhere specific it is mostly in the upper outer quadrant of the breast. Half of all women with this condition have pain in both breasts at the same time. The breast feels nodular to the touch and on mammography there is fibroadenosis with or without cysts. (For more discussion of these conditions see pages 116 and 120).

Pre-menstrual pain is cyclical, worst during the few days leading up to a period, is felt most over the outer and upper regions of the breast and may be accompanied by considerable tenderness. This pain comes about because the breast is swollen with blood and tissue fluid before a period, which is perfectly normal in many women. All the symptoms disappear within a few days of menstruation starting. If the pain is very severe, physical activities and sexual relations become unpleasant or impossible. Starting on the Pill or coming off it may improve things but most drug treatments (apart from simple pain-killers such as aspirin) are ineffective.

Axillary breast tissue can sometimes become painful as the bra or arm rubs against it. Some women have quite a large tail of breast tissue extending from the main breast up into the armpit. It can be removed surgically, if it is giving trouble, with no ill effects on the rest of the breast.

Very large breasts can pull on the connective tissue above the breast where it joins the chest wall and cause pain there. Such women have extreme tenderness on finger pressure on the chest wall at the level of the third ribs. Breast reduction may be indicated if the pain is severe.

Duct ectasia (see also page 118) produces pain too but with no specific time pattern. The pain is often worse in cold weather and the site of the pain is precisely located. Pain under the areola, nipple and inner quadrants of the breast are often caused by this condition. Mammography helps to make the diagnosis.

The *Tietze syndrome* is a condition of the chest wall underneath the breast but produces pains which seem to come from the breast. There is a painful, tender, enlarged rib joint where it joins the breastbone. There is no pattern to the pain and it is very longlasting. The pain is always well localized to the affected joint or joints and doesn't affect the breast itself at all. No one knows what causes this strange condition but the fact that it occurs so rarely in males and does not show up on X-rays of the ribs suggests that it might be directly related to the presence of breast tissue. There is, unfortunately, no satisfactory treatment for the Tietze syndrome.

Trauma is another cause of breast pain. The pain is fairly obviously localized to the site of the injury or to a previous operation scar. The site of previous biopsies or incisions for draining breast abscesses can cause pain at a much later date. Pain is more common if the incision runs radially out from the nipple. Most surgeons like to make incisions that run in the natural skin lines of the breast, which are concentric with the circumference of the areola.

Another common cause of trauma is a poorly fitting bra. Too tight a bra or one with too much uplift can cause breast pain, as can one with wires that dig into the breast. Recently a condition known as 'joggers' nipple' has become the subject of medical interest. This arises in women who jog without a bra (and also in men). The nipples become painful (especially in cold weather when they are more erect) as they rub repeatedly against the inside of the teeshirt, causing soreness of the skin. This troublesome condition can be overcome by covering the nipples with petroleum jelly or some other similar lubricant (talc is also very good) or by wearing a bra or a blouse with a smooth finish (silk or synthetic).

Another common traumatic experience is lovemaking. Some women enjoy very vigorous stimulation of their breasts and nipples, even to the point of considerable pain. Intense squeezing, pinching or biting can cause pain but it usually disappears quickly afterwards. Any masochistic pursuits that really hurt or damage the breast will, of course, be painful but these should be discouraged because of the real danger that the breast could be permanently damaged. *Knocks, blows, love play and other trauma do not, however, cause cancer.*

Cancer is an uncommon cause of breast pain. In one survey pain was the first symptom in only one in ten of all breast cancers. Pain, when it does occur, is localized to the site of the tumour and is usually noticed when the area over the lump is knocked accidentally.

Emotional causes of breast pain can occur but are usually diagnosed only in the absence of any other disease. Such a pain can be anywhere in the breast and of any type. Some experts claim that such women (with no underlying cause for their pains) have more sexual problems than average, poorer marriages and a stronger than normal fear of cancer. Reassurance is usually all that these women need, though underlying marital and personality problems should of course be treated when they are the main problem.

Cervical or dorsal root syndromes can cause pain in the breast. Conditions affecting the cervical (neck) vertebrae or those of the upper back can produce pain in the breast and arm.

Pregnancy produces breast pain in some women. Rarely, pain can be the first sign that a woman is pregnant.

Sore or cracked nipples, blocked ducts, engorgement and breast infection all cause pain and these are discussed on pages 69, 80, 67 and 81 respectively in the chapter on breastfeeding. *The let-down reflex* is also painful for some women (see page 47).

The contraceptive pill can cause breast pain, but this disappears on stopping the Pill. Some women with cyclical mastalgia are improved by taking the Pill. Treatment is often a matter of trial and error.

Cold weather commonly causes quite severe pain in the nipples of some women. Warm clothes are the obvious answer to this problem.

The nature of any given breast pain can often help to point to the diagnosis. The pain in fibrocystic disease (cyclical mastalgia) is cyclical and described as 'full of milk'. This description also applies to Pill pains. Pains arising from the spine are 'sharp and radiating'; those from the Tietze syndrome, 'aching'; from trauma, 'sore', 'bruised' or 'stabbing'; from infections, 'throbbing'; and from duct ectasia, 'itching, burning, or drawing'.

Treatment depends entirely on making the right diagnosis because there are no generalized treatments for breast pain: the specific conditions causing it must be treated. Diuretic drugs (that make a person pass more urine) have been used to cure the supposed water retention that was thought to be the cause of many diffuse and otherwise inexplicable breast pains, but very recent studies show that there is no difference in the total body water levels of those women with and those without breast pain. Various hormonal treatments have also been shown to be no more effective than a placebo in several studies.

Bromocriptine, a drug which lowers blood levels of the hormone prolactin, *is* proving useful in the treatment of some cases of breast pain, especially in those that are cyclical. One study showed an improvement in 75 per cent of the women treated in this way. Danazol, a drug first used in the treatment of endometriosis, is also being used with some success. One study was successful in abolishing pain and nodularity of the breasts in 80 per cent of women. Tenderness responded within one month of treatment but nodules took much longer to go.

Really severe pain that doesn't respond to any other treatment may have to be treated by doing a subcutaneous mastectomy and then replacing the breast tissue with an implant (see page 179). This operation is, however, rarely necessary for breast pain.

Overall, then, the outlook for women who have pain in the breast is better than it has been and is improving. The unsatisfactory results of treatment in the past are hardly surprising because all painful breasts were then treated in the same way. A better understanding of the underlying causes has enabled doctors to tailor-make the treatment to fit the woman.

Breast injuries

The breasts are so prominent and vulnerable that it is surprising that they aren't injured more than they are. That they are not is probably because they are instinctively proteced by a woman when she is threatened with physical danger to the area. Most accidental injuries occur when the woman doesn't have time to put her hands or arms over her breasts in a reflex action.

Fat and blood vessels are in plentiful supply in the breasts so it's hardly surprising that trauma to the breast can cause haemorrhage and fat necrosis (death of fat cells). A tender lump follows quickly after a blow as blood leaks out of local vessels. This blood is walled off and absorbed over the next few weeks and the breast returns to normal. Fat necrosis may produce a hard mass that can later be mistaken for cancer. Except with sharp injuries (knife wounds, for example) no damage is done to the breasts' milk-producing system so breastfeeding is rarely jeopardized because of an old injury.

Although breast injuries cause a hard lump (of blood clot) which can be mistaken for a cancer, they do not *cause* cancer in themselves. It's always difficult to know what to do about a lump that doesn't disappear within a month for example after a knock, but it's probably safest to have it biopsied simply because the knock may have occurred over a pre-existing lump. Many women on discovering a breast lump try to explain it away as the result of a previous injury to the area but often they are doing this subconsciously in an effort to arrive at a less serious diagnosis.

Injuries that occur during lovemaking have been discussed already on page 107.

Burns, scalds (especially from a shower head that spurts hot water unexpectedly), and bashes from toddlers and active young children can all be especially unpleasant on this sensitive area of the body. Burns are particularly painful on the breasts and take a long time to heal. Sunburn can also be very painful on the breasts.

Breast infections

Breast infections are uncommon in women who are not lactating. For a discussion of these infections, see page 80.

Newborn infants of either sex can, rarely, get a breast abscess in the first few days after birth when they are producing 'witch's milk'. See page 124 for details.

Boils, carbuncles and pimples on the breast rarely cause infection of the breast tissue itself. The best treatment for boils anywhere is to incise them and so let the pus out. Squeezing spots or boils can drive the infection from the superficial layers of the skin into the deeper tissues of the breast and so cause mastitis.

Rarely today generalized infections such as TB spread to involve the breast just as they can involve any organ of the body.

Any breast infection can cause the lymph nodes in the armpit to swell. If ever these glands do swell it's wise to tell your doctor.

Nipple problems

Most women have two nipples, one on each breast, but extra nipples are fairly common, occurring in 1 or 2 per cent of all newborn babies. *Supernumerary nipples* are discussed in more detail on page 37 and are probably the commonest congenital abnormality of the nipples. They can easily be removed but many people don't bother.

Very rarely a complete breast is absent (amastia) in which case there is no nipple on that side either. Later on in life a new breast can be made using a silicone implant (see page 203) and a new nipple constructed using some of the areola from the other breast or skin from the vulva (which is the same colour as areolar skin).

Inverted nipples are fairly common. In this condition the nipples, rather than pointing out, are flat or actually indented to form a pit at the centre of the areola. Women with this minor deformity often don't bother to do anything about it, even though sexual gratification from the affected nipple (s) is often poor. They do begin to worry though when they become pregnant and want to breastfeed. Inverted nipples themselves are not dangerous and simply need to be kept clean. Dirt and cellular debris can collect in the pit if it isn't washed thoroughly but this rarely causes problems.

For details of how to manage inverted nipples if you want to breastfeed, see page 65.

Surgery for inverted nipples can be successful but often involves severing all the milk ducts which in this condition tend to be shorter than normal. There is new evidence that even once the nipple has been completely severed at such an operation breastfeeding is sometimes possible as the ducts seem to recanalize in some women.

Inflammation (dermatitis) of the nipples is not uncommon and sometimes occurs as a result of rubbing against rough clothes, after biting during lovemaking, or when breastfeeding. Some women get contact dermatitis (allergic contact dermatitis or contact eczema) if they are sensitive to some ingredient in perfume, bubble bath, powder, or any other preparation used on the nipple skin. Avoidance of the offending substance usually cures this condition within days but sometimes a steroid cream may be necessary. Traces of detergent and fabric softener left in the material or a bra after inadequate washing are another cause of this kind of inflamation. Sometimes sore nipples while breastfeeding are infected with thrush. This needs special treatment. The nipples may also be affected by eczema just as can any other part of the body.

A condition known as Paget's disease of the nipple can look like dermatitis but is much more serious. It is a skin ulceration or inflammation of the nipple secondary to an underlying duct cancer. This type of nipple trouble doesn't clear up and the skin must be biopsied to search for cancer cells. Any unexplained nipple inflammation that doesn't heal after taking simple measures must be biopsied just in case there's trouble underneath. The outlook for Paget's disease, if caught early, is very good.

Nipple retraction occurs when an underlying tumour becomes fixed to the underside of the nipple and draws it inwards. Any nipple retraction or loss of mobility of the nipple calls for immediate medical attention. *Duct ectasia* (see page 118) can also cause nipple retraction.

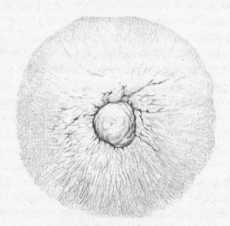

Nipple retraction.

Polyps frequently occur on the skin of the nipple. They take the form of a small rounded head on a stalk and are quite harmless. They can be anything from ½ – 2 cm (⅕ – ¾ inch) long. They rarely give any trouble except that they're a nuisance as they rub on the inside of a bra. They can be quickly and easily removed under a local anaesthetic in an out-patient department.

Papillomas too are harmless growths of the nipple. These tumours start in the nipple's ducts and can be removed under a general anaesthetic. There is little or no scarring as a result of the operation which clears up the condition once and for all.

Odd-looking nipples are common. While most women have cylindrical nipples that sit in the middle of their areolae and point in the same axis relative to the breast itself, some women have strange-looking nipples that are nevertheless perfectly normal. Some women (or more likely their men) worry because their nipples are flat most of the time. This really doesn't matter because the vast majority of such nipples become erect when cold or with sexual stimulation. If you are in any doubt as to whether your nipples are normal, don't hesitate to see your doctor. There's no point worrying when he could easily put your mind at rest. (For more details of normal nipple variations, see page 41.

Nipple discharge occurs very commonly. In fact the normal non-lactating breast produces fluid all the time. As it emerges at the nipple it dries up and is lost. This normal discharge is sometimes slightly more obvious and can stain the inside of the bra a little.

Nipple discharges can be broadly grouped into two types, physiological and pathological. Physiological discharges are almost always bilateral (affect both breasts); arise from many ducts on the nipples; and are easily produced by manual expression or suction. The most obvious member of this group is breast milk, the commonest type of nipple discharge. Similar discharges occur in women who are taking oestrogens, certain tranquillizers (the phenothiazines), some anti-hypertensive drugs, some tri-cyclic antidepressants, and the oral contraceptives. All these drugs can produce an abnormal milk flow by stimulating prolactin secretion. This production of milk in a non-lactating woman can be distressing enough but in a man it is even more troublesome. The occurrence isn't dose-related but does seem to occur more readily with large doses of certain tranquillizers. Many of these drugs can also produce a loss of periods in women and a loss of sex drive in men and some cause breast enlargement in men too. Withdrawal of the drug results in a complete return to normal within a few weeks but if the Pill has been the precipitating cause then the results take longer.

Another type of physiological discharge that can occur is a blood-stained one during pregnancy. This discharge subsides without treatment following delivery of the baby. In some women who have recently had their womb removed and in many women near the menopause, firm squeezing of the areolar area and nipple results in the appearance of a drop or two of a cloudy, milky, thick, greyish secretion.

Pathological nipple discharges in contrast are persistent, though not necessarily continuous and are usually secondary to an underlying pathological condition. Such discharges arise from a single duct on the nipple and often occur from one breast only.

There are five types of pathological nipple discharge. Often the type of discharge helps the doctor decide on the cause, so it's worth noting and telling him in some detail. Remember that the vast majority even of pathological nipple discharges are caused by benign conditions. In women over fifty, though, cancer is the commonest cause of a nipple discharge and must be taken seriously. When cancer is the cause of the discharge there is almost always a lump in the breast as well, even though the woman herself may not be able to feel it. *The combination of a discharge and a lump always calls for a biopsy.*

A milky discharge sometimes occurs during pregnancy and always after childbirth. Milk production continues for as long as a baby is being put to the breast and may not stop for many months after weaning. It may also occur when taking certain drugs (see page 113) or if a woman has a high prolactin level for any reason. Treatment for the latter is basically medical (as opposed to surgical) and may involve giving large doses of oestrogens to suppress the pituitary gland, bromocriptine to lower prolactin levels, or clomiphene citrate. Of course, if a drug or the Pill is the cause, then the treatment is to stop these medications.

A sticky discharge is usually a sign of duct ectasia (see page 118). It is often multicoloured and is sometimes associated with redness, burning pain, itching, and swelling of the nipple and areola. The discharge may look bloody and it is always sticky. If you touch your areola when you have a discharge like this you'll find that it feels like a collection of worms beneath the surface. If this disease progresses untreated the area under the areola becomes hardened with fibrous tissue and then forms a lump which feels like a cancer. This cause of nipple discharge is most common in women near the menopause.

In the early stages scrupulous nipple cleaning and a course of oestrogens will clear it up. For more about the treatment of duct ectasia, see page 118.

A discharge of pus can occur with mastitis caused by infection (for more details see page 80.

A *watery discharge* without any colour is rare. It often suggests an underlying malignancy and a surgeon will want to investigate the cause.

A *bloody or serous discharge* is pale yellow, has a pink tinge or is frankly reddish-brown. Twenty-five years ago it was always said that a bloody discharge was caused by cancer but today we know that such a discharge is usually caused by a benign condition. The commonest causes are an intraduct papilloma (see page 117), fibrocystic disease (page 119) and, less commonly, cancer and advanced duct estasia (page 118). It is also sometimes seen during pregnancy and soon after childbirth. Over the age of fifty a bloody or serous discharge usually means cancer. Most experts think that the breasts of any woman with such a discharge should be explored surgically to rule out an underlying cancer.

It's often difficult even for a doctor to decide whether a nipple discharge is significant or not. By and large, significant ones usually involve one breast only, come from one duct on a nipple, and are not linked to breastfeeding. Some conditions of the breasts and nipples produce a pseudo-discharge which comes from the nipple skin rather than from the ducts. These include eczema of the nipple; inverted nipples; traumatic ulcers (love bites etc); and cold sores. As increasing numbers of women examine themselves each month and become more used to handling their breasts they also become more aware of their normal nipple secretions. Until they realize or are told that these *are* normal many women worry a lot, usually quite unnecessarily.

A nipple discharge then is something to be taken seriously but not necessarily something to worry about. Unless there is a very obvious cause, always see your doctor who will refer you to a specialist if it seems appropriate.

Benign (non-cancerous) conditions of the breast

Contrary to popular belief, the vast majority of breast lumps are *not* cancer — they are benign. This doesn't mean that they don't cause problems or that they should be ignored. Even if you have had a benign breast lump in the past, it's always worth taking a new lump seriously, so see your doctor if you find one. Approximately 80 per cent of all breast lumps are harmless.

A *fibroadenoma* is a very common lump composed of fibrous and glandular tissue. It is the second commonest benign breast condition after fibrocystic disease, which we shall consider below. Fibroadenomas occur most frequently in young adult women but are also the commonest lumps found in girls and teenagers. There is no particular preference for either breast and the condition affects both breasts in one in eight affected women. One in five women with the condition has more than one such lump in the breast.

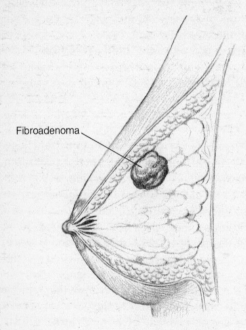

Fibroadenoma

A fibroadenoma.

Such lumps are firm, solid, very mobile and difficult to grasp hold of. They most often occur in the upper outer quadrant of the breast and are easy to feel because of their well-defined edge. Because they seem to be loose within the breast, they have been called 'breast mice': as you try to grasp them they run away from your fingers. They vary considerably in size from about 1 – 5 cm (½ – 2 inches) in diameter, but rarely they become enormous. Usually though they grow very slowly. The cause is not known.

As the diagnosis is usually so straightforward tests are rarely needed and the fibroadenoma is removed surgically by a simple, short operation.

As far as we know, fibroadenomas don't become malignant if left untreated. They are removed because they grow large if left and can deform the breast outline and indeed its tissue. The woman is out of hospital in a few days.

Many women become very emotional and concerned about any breast lump even when they are assured that it is harmless, and it can take such a woman days or even weeks to settle down to her normal life again, even though the lump is not a cancer.

An *intraduct papilloma* is a warty growth within one of the ducts of the breast and is most frequently seen in patients in their forties. The main symptom is a nipple discharge which is either watery, serous, bloody or even greenish, coming spontaneously from a single duct. There is often no lump to be felt although there may be a small non-tender, pea-sized mass beneath the nipple. When a doctor examines you for this problem he'll press all around the circumference of the nipple and when there is a discharge he'll know he's pressed on the lesion. Some women complain of a sensation of fullness or pain in the nipple or areolar area which is relieved when the fluid is expelled by pressure over the affected duct.

No tests are usually necessary to make the diagnosis although some hospitals look at a drop of the discharge under a microscope for cancer cells.

Intraduct papillomas are usually benign but may be pre-cancerous so they are always worth removing. At the operation the surgeon makes an incision 2.5 cm (1 inch) long around the areola where it joins the breast skin. The nipple is then flapped back to show up the ducts underneath. The papilloma is located and removed. If on inspection the surgeon finds other papillomas or duct disease, he removes the whole duct system but this is rarely necessary. The nipple is stitched carefully back into place and the breast looks perfectly normal.

The pathologist examining the removed papilloma will take considerable care to look for cancer cells and if any are found the woman will have to have a simple mastectomy (see page 178). Once you have had an operation for one duct papilloma you are more likely than other women to develop another so you'll be asked to see your surgeon for regular checkups.

Lipomas can occur anywhere on the body and the breast is no exception. A lipoma is a painless lump made up of fat cells. The whole mass is surrounded by a thickened capsule and is thereby easily distinguished from the rest of the breast (much of which is composed of fat anyway). This kind of lump often doesn't show up on X-rays or with other diagnostic tests but is usually easily diagnosed clinically.

A lipoma can be left untreated with no danger to the woman but as it may grow and change the breast size and shape, it is best removed unless it is very small. The operation is simple and involves only a few days in hospital.

A *cystosarcoma phylloides* is an uncommon breast lump but it can grow to a gigantic size quite quickly. It is usually seen in one breast only and in the young rather than the old. On feeling the lump it is firm and rubbery but as it enlarges it can become knobbly. This growth is essentially benign but it can spread to distant organs and can recur locally after removal so it is always taken seriously and removed completely at an operation. If malignant change (which is very rare) is found, the whole breast will have to be removed, otherwise the lump itself is simply removed.

Duct ectasia is a condition in which the ducts inside the breast dilate and become distended with cellular and glandular breakdown products. The main symptom is a nipple discharge but unlike that seen with intraduct papillomas this discharge is sticky, multicoloured, comes from many ducts and affects both breasts. Many women with this condition complain of a burning or itching pain around the nipple and areola and there may be worm-like swellings under the areolae. Less commonly there may be actual pain and redness of the areola, pressure on which produces the sticky discharge. As the condition advances, the clinical picture changes. The ducts become fibrosed and shorten as a result. This pulls the nipple inwards and a lump may be felt under the areola.

Duct ectasia is commonest in women over forty but can continue after the menopause. The surgical treatment is often not easy because so much tissue has to be removed. Some surgeons consider removing most of the breast and then reconstructing it to produce a good appearance. Fortunately it is not a common condition and is not pre-cancerous.

Fibrosis (thickening) of the breast is a condition in which fibrous tissue overgrows in various areas. Fibrosis is also a part of the natural ageing of the breast but such changes with age are usually generalized. In younger women patches of fibrous tissue can form and may be difficult to distinguish from a cancer without tests. In women who have lost a lot of weight and in certain women who have pendulous breasts areas of fibrosis can occur in two areas of the breast. The first is under the breast where it joins the chest wall. Not infrequently, a rope-like band of fibrous tissue can be felt there. The second area affected by fibrosis is the upper outer quadrant of the breast. Thickening here is less likely to be of a serious nature if it is the same in both breasts. Don't forget that this area of the breast is also the commonest one for breast cancers so if ever you feel a thickened area, ask your doctor to check you over.

Fat necrosis occurs when fat cells die as a result of injury, ageing, or rapid weight loss. As fatty tissue in the breast dies it is replaced by fibrous tissue. This produces a firm or hard lump, irregular to the touch, that feels very like a cancer. Mammography may be useful because these lumps sometimes have calcium in them which is easily seen on the X-ray. Most surgeons will want to remove such a lump to be on the safe side.

By far the commonest non-cancerous condition affecting the breast is *fibrocystic disease*. One out of six women between thirty-five and fifty will have this condition. Other names that have been used for the condition are lumpy breasts, cystic disease, cystic mastitis and mastitis.

Fibrocystic disease is a condition of younger rather than older women and seems to be linked to the production (or taking) of oestrogens. The lesions (cysts surrounded by fibrous tissue) are small and multiple and affect both breasts at once. Pain and tenderness is the main characteristic of the condition and many women say they feel 'full, as if with milk'. The symptoms are always worst just before a period and tend to get better after this stage in the menstrual cycle.

There are three fairly distinct stages of the disease. The first occurs in the late teens and early twenties and shows up as painful, tender, pre-menstrual swelling, especially of the axillary tail areas of the breasts. The second stage occurs in the late twenties and early thirties. It is now multiple nodules that create the problems. When the hand is slid over the breast it feels as though there are peas under the skin. Specific lumps can occur if an area of fibrosis forms a hard mass. This can be difficult to differentiate from cancer. The third stage is the

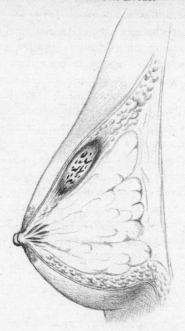

Fibrocystic disease.

cystic phase. When cysts occur there may be a sudden pain, a full feeling, or a burning sensation with the sudden appearance of a lump. The lumps feel cystic (like a soft sorbo rubber ball), are tender, well demarcated and slightly mobile. There may be a discharge from the nipple which is clear, greenish or brown.

When a cyst is diagnosed it is usually aspirated nowadays rather than removed as used to be the practice. A fine needle is used to inject local anaesthetic into the skin over the cyst and then a wider-bore needle is inserted into the cyst while the surgeon holds it steady with his other hand. All the fluid is removed by sucking back up the needle with a syringe and the cyst deflates completely. The amount of fluid withdrawn varies in volume from 5 to 15 ml (up to ½ fl. oz) and in colour from straw to green or brown. Although this is a method commonly used by thousands of surgeons worldwide there are still many who feel that an operation is a safer way of ensuring that a cyst isn't a cancer. This is especially worthwhile if the woman has a family history of breast cancer. Not infrequently a growth is found as well as a cyst. After all, both conditions are common. If after the surgeon has aspirated fluid from a cyst the area has not deflated or if the fluid is bloody, he will usually remove the cyst at an operation, even if he is basically one of the 'aspirating' as opposed to 'operating' surgeons.

Because fibrocystic disease is so unpleasant for many women several non-surgical approaches have been tried. Diuretic drugs have been used pre-menstrually in the hope of reducing the amount of fluid and thereby the tension in the breasts. Male sex hormones too have been tried but with little success. Probably the only useful treatment (other than surgery or aspiration) for definite lumps is to wear a firm, well-fitting bra and to take simple painkillers such as aspirin or codeine when the pain is bad pre-menstrually.

Just why the female breast should be so commonly affected by benign conditions no one knows. We saw in Chapter 1 how modern women's breasts function entirely differently from those of her ancestors so it's quite possible that the answer lies somewhere here. There has recently been a lot of research on whether the Pill has any

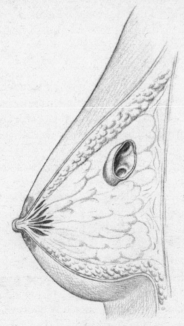

A breast cyst.

effect on benign disease of the breast. There was good reason to assume that by preventing a woman from ovulating while on the Pill her breasts might be more like those of her anovulatory ancestors whose continuous pregnancies and breastfeeding were the cause of their anovulation. This has in fact been borne out in several studies which have found that non-cancerous breast conditions are less common in women who take the Pill. Fibrocystic disease and fibroadenomas especially are less commonly seen. The degree of protection given by the Pill seems to be related to the length of time it is taken. One study found that those women who had taken the Pill for eight years or more had only one-fifth of the benign breast disease of non-Pill women. However, the authors of the study suggest that women with existing benign breast disease should not start taking the Pill. Incidentally, there is no evidence that the Pill causes breast cancer but it does seem to accelerate the growth of existing malignant cells.

From this section we have seen how common benign breast lesions are and how most of them can be easily treated. We shall see how doctors decide whether a lump is a cancer or not in Chapter 7.

CHAPTER 6

The breast at special times of life

In Childhood and adolescence

We saw on page 35 how the breasts develop in the fetus and given that the process is so complicated it is scarcely surprising that abnormalities are relatively common.

Amastia is the name given to the condition in which there is a complete absence of a breast or even both breasts. This comes about because the milk ridge completely regresses in the fetus leaving no breast tissue at all on that side. Persistence of the milk ridge can produce a growth of breast tissue anywhere along its path (the milk line) as described on page 37. Extra or *supernumerary nipples* are fairly common in both sexes. Various studies have found them in between 1

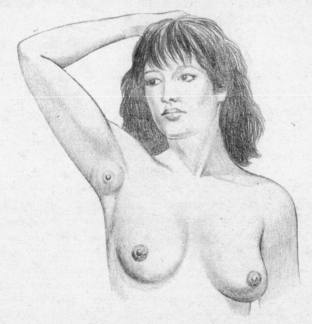

Polymastia — the presence of an extra breast.

and 5 per cent of the population (more often in men). While extra nipples are often seen, true extra breasts are very rare indeed. *Polymastia* is the medical term for extra breasts. When one is present it is usually a simple lump of breast tissue under a supernumerary nipple but rarely it may take the form of a fully developed extra breast that is capable of producing milk.

When a baby is born it is still very much under the influence of its mother's pregnancy hormones that have been transferred via the placental blood supply. Nearly half of all newborn babies of both sexes have some *breast enlargement* caused by these maternal hormones. Some of these breasts actively produce a sort of milk – so-called 'witch's milk' – for a few days. Babies who are breast-fed may continue to have slightly swollen breasts for some months but most babies, whether breast-or bottle-fed, lose their breast swelling within a few weeks at the most. Sometimes the breast of a newborn baby becomes red and tender but true infection rarely occurs.

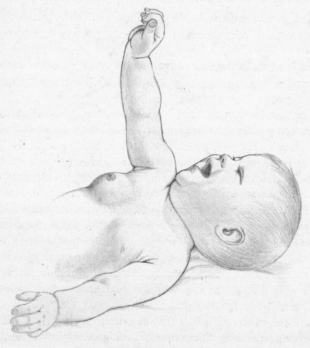

Breast enlargement in a baby.

After this age and until puberty boys rarely have anything wrong with their breasts but girls can start developing breasts prematurely (before puberty) which can be worrying for the parents and a nuisance to the child. It is a common problem. Most girls do not develop any breast tissue before the age of eight or nine but the premature breast development we're talking about here occurs before this age.

The condition is known medically as *premature thelarche* and the degree of development varies enormously. Although some girls' enlarged breasts become small before enlarging again at puberty, most continue to grow steadily and reach full size in adolescence as normal. Both breasts usually enlarge at the same time but they may enlarge separately. No treatment is needed other than to reassure the child and her parents and no tests are necessary. A condition called *precocious puberty* is very much less common. In this the child develops not only breasts but a female shape, pubic and armpit hair, an enlarged clitoris and pigmented areolae, and starts having periods. Girls like this will need a medical examination and some tests just in case the underlying cause for the condition needs to be treated.

The normal development of the breasts at puberty is discussed on page 38.

Gynaecomastia is the name given to any enlargement of the male breast and is discussed on page 236. It is common in pubertal and adolescent boys.

Just as in adult women, the breasts of children and adolescents can develop lumps. About three-quarters of all such breast lumps are *fibroadenomas*. They are much like those in older women (see page 116) but sometimes grow very quickly in adolescent girls. In most girls the tumour is single but one in four affected girls has more than one. No one knows what causes fibroadenomas at any age but they are known to be stimulated by oestrogens. Girls with these lumps don't have any abnormality of their hormones though, so the mystery remains. Most surgeons think it wise to remove these benign lumps mainly because their continued growth can distort the developing breast. Small lumps (which most are) can easily be removed, leaving a hairline scar that is invisible within a year or so. Most adolescent breast lumps occur in late-teenage girls.

A rare pre-cancerous lump that can occur at this age is called a *cystosarcoma phylloides*. These tumours can grow rapidly to reach the size of a small football in a few months. The tumour can easily be excised but rarely the whole breast may have to be removed. Any fast-growing lump in a girl's breast must receive medical attention as soon as possible.

Breast cancer is very rare indeed in girls and adolescents. In fact, fewer than two in a hundred occur under the age of thirty.

Breast enlargement is, however, fairly common. Breasts enlarge anyway in adolescent girls, of course, but in some girls either one or both breasts enlarge dramatically. We have seen already that a harmless fibroadenoma can cause this enlargement, as can a cystosarcoma phylloides. *Virginal hypertrophy* is the term for a diffuse breast enlargement (usually affecting both breasts) that comes on about the time of the first period. Some girls with this harmless, yet worrying, condition have massive breast enlargement and are very embarrassed by it. The enlargement usually occurs over a period of several months and can produce such heavy breasts that back pain and curvature of the spine become a very real problem. Finding clothing and bras becomes very difficult and many of these unfortunate girls end up withdrawing socially. There are no hormone disturbances in such girls and no one knows what causes the problem.

Doctors are very loath to interfere with the developing breast and

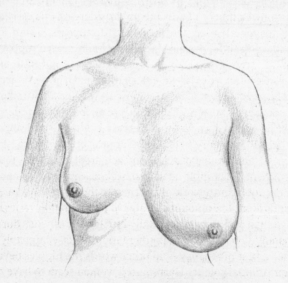

Virginal hypertrophy of the left breast.

will never operate unless they are really concerned. Many mothers are worried because their daughters' breasts are too small or too large but it is rare for a cosmetic surgeon to operate before the age of twenty. Many anomalies seem to correct themselves as the girl goes through adolescence, and surgery done before the age of twenty is often of uncertain outcome.

Sometimes one breast grows faster than the other and indeed may remain bigger throughout a woman's life. Many women have breasts of slightly unequal size and unless there is considerable deformity it's certainly not worth interfering. Any gross difference in size can be very embarrassing for the adolescent girl but it is still better to wait until the adult breast form is complete before considering an operation.

During pregnancy

The breast begins to be affected by pregnancy within a couple of weeks of conception and for many women breast sensations are the first indication that they are pregnant. Some women say that immediately after their first missed period their breasts begin to feel full (as they do pre-menstrually) and within another two or three weeks they begin to feel rubbery and full to an outsider. At this early stage the breasts may be tender but this often disappears within a few weeks. In addition to tenderness there may be increased nipple sensitivity and some tingling. The breasts enlarge slowly and at the end of the sixth week after the last menstrual period they are usually noticeably bigger. The tail of breast tissue that lies up under the armpit in some women is especially liable to become swollen and tender. The superficial veins of the breast begin to swell and tiny lumps (called Montgomery's tubercles) appear on the areola. There are between six and twelve of these on each areola and they may be tender or swollen. The nipple itself also becomes more prominent.

Around the fourteenth week of pregnancy the nipples and areolae begin to get darker. The amount and area of pigmentation varies from woman to woman and anyway is usually much more obvious during a first pregnancy. Once there the pigmentation never completely disappears after a first pregnancy – in other words the nipples never go back to their original colour. Dark-haired women seem to have more pregnancy pigmentation than do fair-haired ones and red-haired

The Breast

women often have very little pigmentation at all. In some women the pigmentation spreads beyond the areola itself and on to the skin of the breast to form a secondary areola. If this occurs it does so at about the eighteenth to twentieth week of pregnancy. Occasionally it can involve much of the skin of the breast. The secondary areola disappears very quickly after delivery in most women. Breastfeeding makes no difference to the permanency of normal pregnancy pigmentation.

Women with small breasts are often delighted by the increase in size that occurs during pregnancy. Those with larger breasts don't notice such a dramatic change in size. Most of this increase in size comes about as a result of glandular growth in the breast but many women also put on a lot of weight during pregnancy. This weight will be distributed all over the body and the breasts will get their share.

Most women say that their breasts are slightly less firm after a pregnancy than they were before it, but it is women who put on a lot of weight who are most likely to get stretch marks and droopy breasts once pregnancy and breastfeeding are over. Wearing a well-fitting, supportive bra in pregnancy and while breastfeeding helps keep your breasts in good shape but this is no substitute for keeping slim. It's also important to prevent engorgement (see page 67) because this can so stretch the breasts as to produce stretch marks and drooping later.

Many women find their breasts become more tender throughout most of pregnancy and as a result they are more sensitive about their breasts being touched and knocked. This can be especially difficult if you have little children who climb all over you and many mothers complain that their toddlers seem to know their breasts are more sensitive than usual because they bash them so much! Lovemaking positions and techniques may need to be modified during pregnancy to reduce the amount of stimulation and foreplay the breasts receive. If your breasts are too tender to be touched tell your partner or show him ways in which they can be caressed so that you both enjoy it. A little care on the part of the man and guidance from you should overcome any such problems.

Most women's nipples become more prominent than usual during pregnancy but some remain flat or actually indented throughout pregnancy. The nipples also become more 'protractile' (elastic) so that the baby can get them well back into his mouth while feeding. Nipple care in pregnancy is discussed on page 64.

From the fifth month or so of pregnancy the breasts may start to leak a few drops of colostrum (early milk) which may be clear or yellowish. This is perfectly normal and is simply the first sign that the breast tissue is starting to produce milk.

Breasts can develop diseases in pregnancy just as at any other time. Unfortunately they are often more difficult to detect during pregnancy because of the swelling and unusual consistency the breasts have at this time. Benign lumps need not be operated on if found late in the pregnancy and can be dealt with after the birth of the baby; but cancers need to be operated on as quickly as usual. In the past it was thought that cancers occurring in a pregnant or lactating breast were very serious and particularly lethal but this has now been shown to be untrue. Breast cancer during pregnancy sometimes produces a red, hot, swollen breast and for this reason it used to be called inflammatory cancer. Fortunately, such a cancer is extremely rare and even when it occurs it does not necessarily mean that the pregnancy will have to be terminated. It used to be thought that the large amounts of oestrogen being produced by the placenta worsened the state of the breast tumour, but several surveys have found this not to be the case and pregnant women with a breast cancer are no longer automatically considered for abortion. To be fair, though, the occurrence of breast cancer among women who are pregnant is so low that very few medical centres have extensive experience of the combination. Perhaps with a better understanding of oestrogen receptors (see page 197) a more positive approach will be taken towards the problem in the future. Women with measurably high levels of oestrogen receptors could be offered an abortion to spare their tumour the effects of placental oestrogen.

Pregnancy is not a contra-indication to radical surgery, if it is needed, and radiation therapy and chemotherapy can be used just as if the woman were not pregnant. Radical surgery and radiation therapy have no adverse affects on the fetus.

As for breast care during pregnancy, if it gives you or your partner pleasure to rub creams into your breasts go ahead and do so but don't expect it to have any permanent effect on the breast once the baby is born. There is no certain preventative for stretch marks apart from not getting too fat. Nipple creams, ointments and sprays are also a waste of time and scrubbing and other methods of 'hardening' the nipples, so beloved of old-style midwives, are not only unpleasant to perform but have no provable value. A healthy woman's nipples need no treatment whatsoever during pregnancy, and no preparation of this sort is necessary for breastfeeding.

During breastfeeding

The breasts undergo more changes while breastfeeding than at any other time during a woman's life. Not only do they start producing large amounts of milk – enough to nourish a baby completely for at least six months, and enough to provide all the water he needs – but they also fluctuate greatly in size many times a day and the appearance of the nipples and the areolae alters.

As the contents and the amount of the first milk produced by the breast – the colostrum – gradually change in the hours after birth, the breasts become much fuller. As the let-down of the milk (see page 47) becomes reliable, the baby will be able to empty the breast of as much milk as he needs each time he is at the breast. Sometimes he'll want a lot of milk and the breast will noticeably change in size from the beginning to the end of a feed. Sometimes he'll only want a few sucks, perhaps as he is going off to sleep, and there'll be no difference in breast size. When a lot of milk is taken off, the mother will notice that her breasts not only look smaller but feel more comfortable and less tense. From time to time, particularly in the early days of breast-feeding, she'll sometimes put her baby to her breast simply to relieve the discomfort from an overfull, tense breast and to prevent engorgement (see page 67) even if the baby isn't actually ready for a feed.

It's interesting that during the months of breastfeeding the breasts often seem to revert slowly to their original, pre-pregnancy size even though they are still producing lots of milk. The breast is at its largest soon after childbirth because the milk supply takes time to adjust to the baby's needs and too much may be produced at first.

Breastfeeding is associated with a further change in nipple shape as the baby's constant sucking makes the nipple skin thicker and more resilient. The increased protractility (see page 128) noticed during pregnancy continues and may increase. Nipple soreness and even cracking may be a problem (see page 69) but can be overcome if you know what to do. The nipples certainly become less sensitive as they toughen up over the weeks and months. After weaning, they will gradually resume their pre-pregnancy state and will become smaller and the skin more sensitive.

The let-down reflex causes characteristic sensations in the breast in many women, though some experience few if any of these sensations though their milk is letting down satisfactorily. The breasts feel warm to the touch because of the enormous increase in blood supply to the whole breast. The nipples erect and may tingle. Milk spurts or leaks out in a series of jets whose timing is specific to each woman. Many women also experience feelings of pleasure as their milk lets down and they may be eager for their babies to suck to relieve the tension in their breasts. The let-down reflex can be inhibited by anxiety and it's important not to cut feeds so short — as is done in many maternity hospitals — that the milk doesn't have a chance to be let down at all.

During and after the menopause

The breast is an important part of a woman's sexual and reproductive system yet as women now live well into their seventies on average, for about a third of their lives their breasts have no reproductive function.

The menopause is a diffuse physiological and psychological phenomenon that happens in women on average at about the age of forty-nine. At this time of life, female hormone secretion from the ovaries diminishes and eventually stops completely. Whether or not the actual glands continue to produce meaningful amounts of sex hormones may well explain why it is that different women seem to suffer from menopausal symptoms in so many different ways.

A cessation of menstruation is the main physiological change that is apparent to a woman and she may in addition have any combination of hot flushes, sweats, depression, irritability, dryness of the skin, itching of the vulval area, dryness of the vagina and certain breast changes.

The breasts of menopausal women change in several ways. During the forties and fifties the amount of glandular tissue gradually diminishes but because there is a compensating increase in fibrous tissue and fat (many women put on weight in their middle years) the breasts may look much the same. As the years pass fat is generally lost from the breasts, the skin becomes more wrinkled and the breasts less full. The natural supporting fibres also tend to weaken a little and the breasts droop more than they did. None of these changes need necessarily make a post-menopausal woman's breasts look unattractive, which is just as well because in today's society women rightly do not see their sexual attractiveness as ending once they cease to be fertile.

With contraception no longer a problem many couples enjoy a better sex life than ever. There is no reason why, given no gross weight changes in either direction, the average woman cannot keep an attractive bust well into her old age. While on the subject of sexuality and the breast at this age it's worth pointing out that many women experience extreme nipple sensitivity during the menopause, though the cause for this is not known. Sometimes this tenderness is accompanied by swelling, redness and enlargement of the nipple. Although these changes are usually normal and completely harmless, it's wise to seek your doctor's opinion. Changes take place in the internal sexual organs too – the uterus shrinks to about 2½ centimetres (1 inch) from top to bottom and the vaginal part ceases to be felt in the vagina. The lining of the uterus (the endometrium) becomes a thin layer with few cells and the muscle of the uterus is gradually replaced by fibrous tissue. The vagina narrows, the labia shrink, and there is some loss of pubic hair. A woman's sex drive may or may not be reduced and weight gain is common.

Many of these symptoms can be prevented or reversed by the taking of oestrogen tablets but a book such as this is no place to discuss such a controversial issue. Whatever the advantages of such therapy, there may be long-term disadvantages. Nature meant post-menopausal women to be low in oestrogens and meddling with the system could well do harm. Synthetic hormones are powerful chemicals and even though many women are obsessed with keeping youthful-looking breasts they must weigh the potential hazards of long-term oestrogen therapy against the small cosmetic gains. Plastic surgery on the breasts can, however, be carried out safely after the menopause and is increasingly being done. Some older women with very pendulous breasts get great physical relief from such surgery.

As women get older their statistical chances of developing breast cancer increase. This means that every woman past the menopause should continue to feel her breasts for lumps and should be examined by a doctor at least once a year. As an older woman's breasts get less fatty it becomes easier to feel lumps, so they can be detected earlier and possibly cured more successfully. Not every breast lump after the menopause is a cancer, of course, and benign conditions still occur. Any nipple discharge, especially if it is bloody, should be reported to a doctor who will then examine the breasts thoroughly. Unfortunately, a nipple discharge often means cancer when it occurs after the menopause. Similiarly, any ulcers of the nipple should be reported to a doctor at once. Having said this, though, with today's safe surgery the outlook for older women who develop breast cancer is very good and is certainly not dramatically worse than that for younger women. On the contrary, it is thought that cancers grow more slowly in the elderly.

CHAPTER 7

Detecting disease

In this chapter we'll look at the detection of disease in the breast. The majority (about 90 per cent) of breast disease is first discovered by a woman herself so let's start by looking at self-examination of the breasts.

Self-examination

Few methods of disease detection can be so appealing as that of breast self-examination. It is simple, costs nothing and is entirely without danger. There is also no doubt that discovering tumours (cancers or malignant lumps) early saves lives. However, millions of women in the Western world, scared into doing something to detect early breast cancer, often don't know exactly what to do and so may well be wasting their time and lulling themselves into a false sense of security while a feelable lump grows in their breast. There are considerable problems with self-examination of the breast, though, so it isn't simply a matter of teaching a woman and then assuming that she'll keep on doing it. Many women have a fear or dislike of examining their own breasts, partly because of what they might find and partly because they see their breasts as 'no-go' areas of their body and are not at ease with handling them. This is not difficult to understand. After all, how many men would take their underpants down in front of a mirror each month and carefully examine their testicles for tumours?

By and large doctors are more successful at discovering breast lumps than are women themselves but as we have already seen, the vast majority of lumps are detected by the women who have them, often quite by chance. One study found that of those practising regular self-examination only 60 per cent discovered their tumour by this method.

Well over 100,000 new cases of breast cancer are discovered each year in the USA and for those women whose tumour is small (less than 1 cm or ½ inch across) the chances of survival are 80 to 90 per cent. However, even with statistics such as these being made known to women through the popular press the average woman still waits five to six months before reporting her lump to a doctor. This procrastination may well allow early treatable disease to spread and such spread undoubtedly reduces the woman's prospect of survival.

We have already seen that the likelihood of any breast lump being a cancer is small (benign lumps account for four-fifths of all lumps) but as a woman gets older the odds increase that a lump will be a cancer. A lot of work has been done on the rate at which cancer cells reproduce and calculations based on this research have shown that by the time a breast cancer can be felt (becomes palpable) it has been there for between two and eight years already. It is very difficult to feel a lump of less than 1 cm diameter (about the size of a marble) except in the very smallest breasts, and much larger tumours can go undetected for many more years, especially in large, pendulous breasts. This means that a tumour first found by a woman in her late thirties could have been there since her late twenties and could have been treated earlier. Surely this is a good reason for every woman to learn how to examine her breasts right from her early twenties.

Learning to examine your breasts may not come easily to you and you may want to get your partner to read this section so that he can do it for you. Many women learn about breast self-examination very sketchily and then worry whether their ability to detect disease amounts to anything. Very often it doesn't.

Before going any further it probably makes sense to re-read Chapter 2 ('What Breasts Are and What They Do') because then you can imagine what you are feeling. When you are learning to feel your breasts it can all be very confusing but after a few weeks you'll be amazed at how expert you've become. All the normal structures in the breast, including the glands and the fat, feel soft and granular to the touch. Being able to distinguish these is a skilful business, even for a trained doctor, so don't expect too much. The vast majority of lumps that matter though feel very different from normal breast tissue, so with practice you're unlikely to confuse the two. The secret of success is to examine your breasts regularly each month immediately after a period *so you are totally familiar with what they feel like normally*. If there's any change at all you'll then notice it quickly.

So as to become expert at knowing what you're feeling you can train yourself in some simple ways. First, close one eye and place a fingertip on an eyelid. Gently move the finger and so slide the eyelid over the underlying eyeball. The eye feels slippery and movable with the lid sliding easily over it. This is what a breast cyst would feel like. Next, pick up your eyelid and lift it away from the eyeball. It comes away easily.

Now place your fingertips on the end of your nose and try to move the skin of the nose without moving the tip of your nose. You won't be able to do it. Also you won't be able to pick up the skin of the nose tip either. This is very much how a serious lump will feel in your breast. If ever you feel a firm (like the nose tip) lump which is attached to the skin, consult your doctor at once.

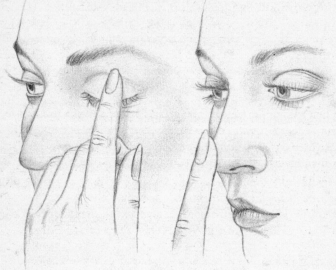

A useful exercise to get used to feeling different textures. The skin moves freely over the 'cyst-like' eyeball but is fixed to the 'cancer-like' nose.

Now that you have the basic 'feels' right, let's look at another training exercise before you go ahead with feeling for lumps. With the pads of two or three fingertips run over the skin on the back of your hand. This enables you to feel the skin but very little underneath. Next, press the skin with your fingertips and move the skin over the tendons underneath. Rotating your fingertips gently in circular patterns, move all over the back of your hand feeling everything as you go. You'll soon build up a pretty accurate picture of the structures underneath. As you get the feel of this remember never to dig your fingertips or nails into yourself when examining your breasts. The most sensitive parts of the fingertips are the flat surfaces, not the ends.

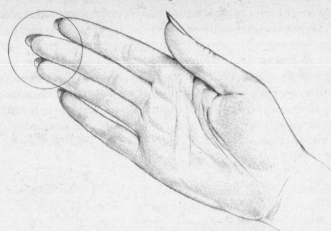

The finger *tips* are used to feel for lumps.

When it comes to routine breast examination, all you need is a large mirror and ten minutes a month. If you are pre-menopausal the best time to do the examination is immediately after your period. If you are post-menopausal (or have had your ovaries removed) do it on a fixed day each month.

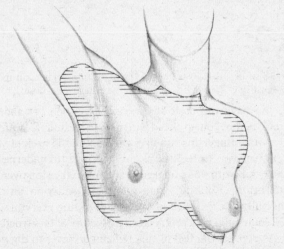

Breast tissue can occur in any part of the cross-hatched area so all of this should be examined each month as well as the breasts.

Try if you can to examine your breasts at the same time of day on each occasion. There are three stages.

Stage 1. *The mirror test.* First stand in front of a mirror with your breasts bare. Look carefully at them. Very few women are symmetrical, so don't worry if your breasts are of different sizes. All you need to do is to look carefully to see if your breasts are any different from normal.

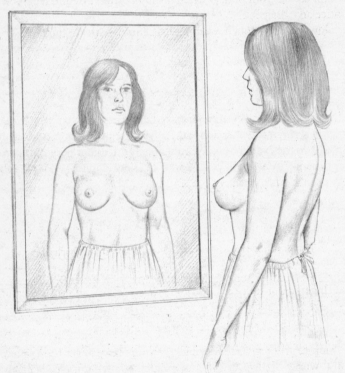

Looking at your breasts in the mirror is an essential part of every monthly examination.

Stand with your arms at your sides. Is one breast bigger than the other? Is one lower than the other? Are the contours round and smooth or are there dimples or bulges that change their outline? Does each nipple point in the same axis as its breast?

If you were to draw an imaginary line through the centre of the nipple in the direction in which the nipple points this would be called the nipple axis. It is usually different for both breasts. See what is normal for you and look for any change from this.

Are both nipples equally erect or does one stay flat or even turned in? Is there anything special about the skin of the breast? Are there any moles, rashes, eczema or dimpling?

Once you have done this, change your position in relation to the mirror so that your breasts catch the light differently and see if you can notice anything else.

Now you can touch your breasts. Start with the *nipples*. Try to

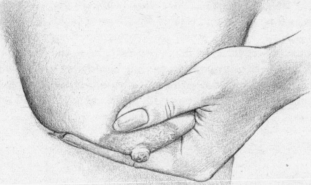

The position of the hand when looking for nipple discharge.

express some secretion from the nipples by pressing with the sides of the fingers. For more details of nipple secretions and their meaning, see page 113. Make a habit of looking at the inside of your bra cups to see if there is any staining from nipple discharge.

Look next for inverted nipples. If yours have never been pointed, don't worry. However, if a normally pointed nipple changes to become flat or even inverted, then this could be caused by a tumour and needs medical attention. As there are non-cancerous causes for nipple inversion, there's no need to worry unnecessarily.

Inspect your nipples for sores, ulcers and eczema. Any ulcer or sore that goes on for more than two weeks should be seen by a doctor.

Some women have symmetrical or mirror image dimples in both breasts within the pigmented area of the areola. These are usually quite normal on the lateral (outer) side below the nipple, but any change in them can indicate disease. When you feel the nipple and areola don't be alarmed because the breasts feel more granular here. The milk ducts are often easily felt as slippery and movable under the areola.

The skin of the breasts is usually like that of the rest of the body. Some women have quite prominent veins on their breast skin, but again there is no cause for concern if this is normal for you. Any new veins should be reported to your doctor. These veins are easily visible in pregnancy, during lactation and in some women on the Pill, and also during the second two weeks of the menstrual cycle.

Orange-peel skin is one important sign to look for when examining your breasts in the mirror. Whenever a lymph duct becomes blocked the tissue fluid that would usually drain down it builds up and makes the skin swell. The area of skin involved becomes raised, swollen and firm and the pores enlarge. This appearance is just like skin-coloured orange peel. It is always worth reporting this finding to your doctor.

Patches of redness are worth looking for too. These can be a sign of inflammation or infection, especially if the area is warm and tender.

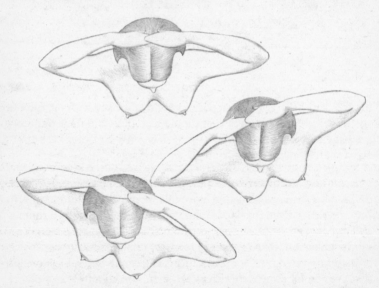

Some positions to adopt in front of a mirror. Moving from side to side enables you to see breast changes more easily.

Tell your doctor about it.

Moles and freckles are commonly seen on the breasts but usually cause no problems. If they occur on any part of the skin where your bra rubs it is probably wise to have them removed because long-standing irritation of a mole can make it turn malignant.

When you have looked for all of these things, raise your arms, place your hands behind your head and as the skin of the breasts tightens see if any new signs appear. Sometimes a bulge or a dimple will occur over an underlying lump when the position of the breasts is altered. Another good way of looking for this sort of change is to bend forwards from the waist and to let your breasts hang down under gravity. Look in the mirror for any change.

Stage 2: Feeling your way around. This stage should ideally be done standing up. Most women find that standing in a shower or in the bath is the best place for this part of the palpation (the medical word for feeling) of their breasts. Thoroughly cover your breasts with soap and examine each breast with the opposite hand (the right breast is

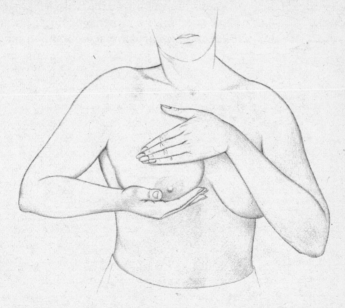

The position of the hands when examining the breasts under a shower.

examined with the left hand and the left breast with the right hand), keeping the hand on the same side as the breast you're feeling behind your neck as you feel with the opposite hand. This works well for women with small breasts but if they are medium or large you'll need to use both hands. To do this, lift the breast with the hand on the same side and let it lie there as if on a shelf. With the other hand feel the top surface of the breast, then hold the top hand steady and feel the underneath of the breast with the bottom hand. Repeat the procedure for the opposite side. Be sure to feel not only the actual breast itself but also the surrounding areas. Many women have breast tissue up into the armpit, high on the chest wall, or even below the breast itself. Lastly, feel the whole breast between your two hands.

The secret of good breast self-examination is to be systematic about it. It really doesn't matter what your system is as long as you work one out and stick to it. The idea is to cover the whole area from the collarbone to below the breasts and up into the armpits.

Most women find it easier to start at the 12 o'clock position and then travel around the breast in a circle working clockwise. Start with the outer edge of the breast area and go all around the clock. When you're back at 12 o'clock move your fingers a couple of finger-breadths towards the nipple and repeat the circular examination. Repeat this

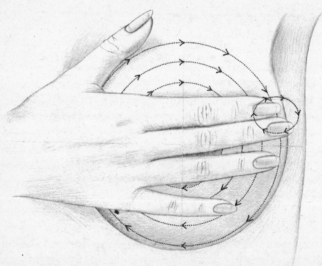

The way to work around the breast systematically with the fingertips.

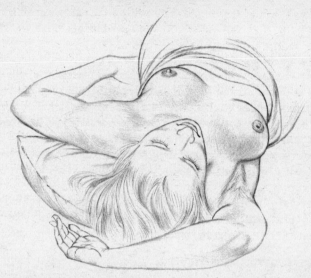

By placing a pillow under the shoulder on the side to be examined the breast sits flat on the chest wall and is easier to examine.

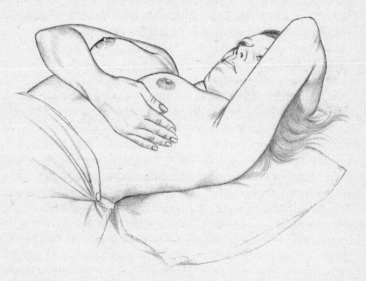

Don't forget to feel right to the outer edges of the breasts and up under the armpits.

until you arrive at the nipple. You will have already examined this when looking in the mirror so you won't need to touch it now.

Stage 3: Examining your breasts lying down. Once you've completed the circular patterns lie down on a firm surface and place a small pillow or a towel under your shoulder on the side to be examined. This raises that side of the chest so that the breast becomes horizontal (instead of falling over the edge of the chest). Some experts suggest feeling your breasts in this position through a piece of sheeting or thin towelling because, they argue, it helps immobilize the skin with the fingertips and allows a better feel of the deeper structures. This is, however, entirely optional.

With the pillow underneath and your hand on that side behind your neck or head, proceed as above, feeling in concentric circles for lumps between your fingertips and your chest.

WHAT YOU MIGHT FIND

1. *Thickened areas.* Some women with heavy breasts and those who have recently lost weight may be able to feel thickened areas immediately under the breasts where they join the chest wall and in the upper outer quadrant of the breast. These thickenings are usually bilateral (present in both breasts) but if they occur on one side only it's worth consulting your doctor.

2. *Normal lumps.* Many women, especially if they have the very common condition known as fibrocystic disease (see page 119), have lumpy breasts most of the time. Get to know your breasts really well so that you can tell when a new lump appears. If you have any doubts, ask your doctor.

3. The *chest wall* is easily felt unless you have very large breasts. You can feel the breastbone, the joints where the ribs join the breastbone, floating ribs below the breast and the xiphoid cartilage at the bottom of the breastbone itself. All of these structures are quite normal and have nothing whatever to do with breast lumps.

4. *Breast tissue outside the breasts* is not at all uncommon. Many women have a tail of breast extending up into the armpit so making the breast 'comma' shaped. This axillary tail can be found on one side or both and is quite normal. It often becomes swollen and tender just before a period and with pregnancy and lactation. It obviously must be examined regularly just like all other breast tissue.

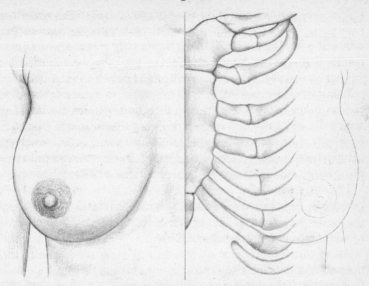

The bones under the breast. Some of these can be felt and misinterpreted as lumps.

5. *Lipomas* are fatty tumours that are sometimes felt in the breast. They are harmless but can feel like a cancer (see page 172). It is often difficult to distinguish these tumours from breast tissue, especially as they are commonly found in the armpits.

6. *A sebaceous cyst* occurs when a skin (sebaceous or oil) gland becomes blocked. Such a lump is fixed to the skin and may be seen to have a tiny pinpoint-sized black duct at the centre.

7. *A lump*. There really is no point trying to be clever about breast lumps. If you find one simply tell your doctor at once and let him make the decision about what should be done. Remember that about eight out of ten of all lumps are not cancerous. Go at once to your doctor, though, because the six-months that most women wait before seeing a doctor moves them from the 80 to 90 per cent long-term cure group to the 40 per cent cure group. Reconstructive surgery is also easier if a tumour is caught early.

Why do women put off going to the doctor? Undoubtedly the main reason is fear. Once a lump is made known to a doctor most women feel that the matter is out of their hands and that they will be placed on a medical merry-go-round over which they have no control. Undoubtedly a good relationship with your doctor is the best start to coping with a breast lump because then you'll have confidence that any action that needs to be taken will be and that unnecessary tests and operations will be avoided.

Many women delay seeking help because they (often wrongly) fear their husband's reaction. Others feel that cancer couldn't possibly happen to them; others are too shy to go for a breast examination; and many women make excuses to themselves about family events, often using every sort of self-deception to put off the actual day.

Finding a breast lump isn't like discovering you have a cold; it's potentially serious and needs dealing with. The earlier you seek help the sooner your mind will be put at rest if it is a harmless lesion and the sooner the treatment can begin if it isn't.

All of this self-examination section may seem very complex and time-consuming but it isn't. Most women become so expert at it that they can do all the things we've outlined in ten minutes a month. That really isn't asking very much when you consider the advantages.

Some women can't bring themselves to touch their breasts for emotional or other psychological reasons. There are two ways around this. Either they can go to their doctor every few months or they can ask their partner to feel their breasts regularly and systematically. Unfortunately, there will always be a proportion of women who will be too lazy or too uneasy about their breasts to do either of these things.

It has been argued that telling women to feel their breasts every month will make them neurotic and self-centred. There is undoubtedly some truth in this because drawing a woman's attention every month to the possibility that she may have a breast lump is bound to have some negative effects. However, as with everything in life we have to compromise and it is generally agreed that the advantages gained from proper self-examination are so great that it is well worth while. Anyway, a woman who is neurotic about breast cancer (or indeed anything else) is unlikely to be tipped into any more serious a psychological state by feeling her breasts each month. Clearly, a woman who is so obsessed with cancer that she examines her breasts every few days is in need of other help.

What a doctor will do

When you go to a doctor complaining of a breast lump he'll examine your breasts in a systematic way rather like that outlined above. He'll begin by feeling in the neck for any enlarged lymph nodes and will feel in the armpits for nodes too. He'll probably examine your breasts with your arms up and then down by your sides and with you sitting and lying down. Some doctors shine a light from a powerful torch through the substance of your breast as you sit in a dark room but this diagnostic method is less commonly used today.

If there is nothing wrong the doctor will tell you and may ask you to feel for yourself so that you can get to know what is normal and what isn't. Now is your opportunity to discuss anything about your breasts with the doctor. Some women go to their doctors complaining of something 'wrong' with their breasts when the real reason is often that they are dissatisfied with their size or something else about them, for example, that they are not symmetrical. No one will think you stupid for raising such questions and fears − after all, why should you automatically know about such things?

We have seen that it makes sense for a woman to examine her own breasts each month but this doesn't mean that she can go for years without seeing a doctor. It still makes sense that post-menopausal women (in whom the risk of breast cancer is higher) should be examined by a doctor twice a year. The breast is a fluctuating organ. A lump may suddenly appear or disappear and this can happen within a very short time of having been pronounced 'clear' by a doctor. Because of this a doctor will often suggest that you return for a repeat examination if he isn't completely happy with what he's feeling. He'll usually ask you to come back at a time half-way between your periods when the breast tissue is at its least active. This makes the job of sorting out the diagnosis that much easier.

BIOPSY AND CYTOLOGY

A biopsy is the removal of a piece of tissue from the body so that it can be examined microscopically by a pathologist. Cytology is the study of cells removed from the body. By studying the nature of the cells in the piece of tissue or the cells in some aspirated fluid, the pathologist can usually diagnose the nature of the disorder.

When a nipple discharge or a lump is discovered, cells in the discharge and cells in the tissue from the lump will be carefully examined, not only to confirm the diagnosis (which might anyway be very clear clinically) but also to help the surgeon plan treatment. Pathologists used to dealing with breast specimens are very accurate in their findings at biopsy and on cytology and extremely rarely make a mistake. This makes these procedures invaluable tools in the hands of a surgeon.

Three types of biopsy are done on breast lumps. The first is an *aspiration biopsy*. At this procedure a doctor puts a little local anaesthetic into the skin over the lump to be biopsied and then inserts a slightly larger and longer needle into the lump. When he pulls back on the syringe to which the needle is attached, some cells and broken-up pieces of tissue are sucked up (aspirated). These are spread on to glass slides ready for staining and microscopic examination. A positive biopsy can be helpful to both patient and doctor because it enables the surgeon to tell the woman before she has her surgery whether she will wake up after the operation with her breast or without it. Without an aspiration biopsy women go into the operating theatre not knowing what the outcome will be and this causes a lot of unnecessary worry. A positive biopsy means that she knows what to expect. A negative finding does not, unfortunately, rule out a cancer. The cancer cells may simply have been missed by the needle. If the result is negative then the lump will be removed at an operation and a frozen section done of the tumour (see page 149) to see whether or not the whole breast should be removed. It has been said that such aspiration or 'needle' biopsies are unhelpful because the woman has to live with the certain knowledge of her cancer before the operation, but on the other side of the coin are the many women who value this time to come to terms with their plight before a serious and psychologically emotive operation is performed.

An *incisional biopsy* is one at which a piece of a lump is cut out at an operation. Under general anaesthesia the lump is biopsied − but only if it is very large. Small and medium-sized lumps are removed complete and then examined microscopically. When the whole lump is removed the procedure is known as an *excisional biopsy*. Very often the lump is examined pathologically while the woman is still under the anaesthetic on the operating table. In this way, if the result comes back positive, the surgeon can go ahead and remove the breast or do whatever else is necessary without the woman having to have a second operation on another day. Because the pathologist freezes the tissue before he cuts (sections) it for examination, this type of procedure is called a 'frozen section'. While frozen-section examinations are very accurate it is necessary for the surgeon to await the final microscopic examination that takes place after the operation before he can tell the woman she is definitely free from cancer (although the pressures are on him to say something at once and most do). In the vast majority of cancers this later result is the same as that obtained under frozen section but a good surgeon will always be cautious about giving a clean bill of health until the final tests are over.

The operations for incisional and excisional biopsy are simple (assuming of course that the lump is non-cancerous and a mastectomy isn't needed). The skin incision is only 5–8 cm (2–3 inches) long in either case and the operation is completed in less than half an hour. Small lumps (less than 3 cm or about an inch in diameter) are often removed completely for examination (especially if they lie centrally within the breast), while larger tumours and those lying at the edge of

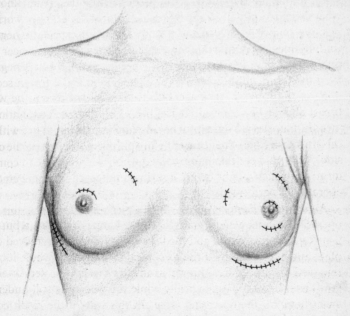

The common positions for breast biopsy scars. Only one incision will be used in any one woman at any given biopsy.

the breast are biopsied using the incisional method. The illustration on page 149 shows the different incisions used for biopsies. Only one will be used at any given biopsy in any one woman, of course.

Today, women are increasingly involving themselves in their treatment and many do not want to give permission for the surgeon to do whatever he wants to if he finds a lump to be a cancer. More and more women are saying something like, 'Do a biopsy, possibly with me as an out-patient, and then we'll discuss the options if the result shows it to be a cancer.' After all, the treatment of breast cancer is by no means simple or agreed upon and women are naturally increasingly unwilling to 'leave it all to the doctors' without a lot of discussion first. If you are in any doubt about what you are signing when asked to sign your consent form before the operation, don't sign it. Ask the nursing sister in charge or one of the doctors to explain what it means.

MAMMOGRAPHY

Mammography is an X-ray technique for examining the breasts. It is used as a method of screening seemingly healthy women for breast lumps and for sorting out the causes when there is a lump. Unfortunately the breasts are difficult to X-ray because the structures inside are very similar in tissue density as shown on X-rays, which work on the principle of showing up one tissue against another by their relative densities to X-rays. Over the last twenty years advances in photographic film technology (all X-rays are recorded on photographic film just as with any other film camera) and equipment have made mammography safe and accurate. One survey found that 97 per cent of breast tumours could be detected by this method though other experts would not put the figure this high.

The most common reason for a woman to have a mammographic X-ray is to help doctors decide whether a lump (found by them or the woman herself) is in fact a cancer. Other women, known to be at a high risk of developing cancer, are also screened from time to time, usually at yearly intervals, so as to pick up any growth early. We shall look at screening for breast cancer at the end of this chapter.

Mammography is a very simple procedure from the woman's point of view. You sit with the breast to be X-rayed on a ledge on which there is an X-ray plate. The radiographer then places a balloon between the breast and the X-ray machine over the breast to compress it and the X-ray is taken just like any other. The compression of the breast helps because it spreads the tissue over a wider area of the X-ray plate, and makes the breast 'thinner'. This makes the picture easier to interpret. Many X-ray units also ask you to lie on your side so that a picture can be taken across the breast as well.

Younger women's breasts are filled with a lot more glandular tissue than are those of older women and this can make reading the X-rays more difficult. Because of this it has often been claimed that mammography is only suitable for older women. This is not true. It is still a very accurate method of detecting cancers in young women and often picks up lumps that can't be felt in these more active and bulky breasts.

Because mammography involves a dose of X-rays, some women are uneasy about having too many of them or even having a once-a-year check-up involving mammography. These fears are understandable but unnecessary. A combination of the early X-ray machines and their films did indeed mean that quite a lot of radiation was used but today this is no longer true. Today's photographic films are so sensitive that very much smaller doses of X-rays are needed and modern equipment delivers the X-rays specifically and selectively to those parts being examined. The days of X-ray machines that spread X-rays all around the room are gone.

Much of the controversy over repeated mammographic X-rays arose because of two reports, in 1965 and 1968. The first concerned patients who had tuberculosis and were being treated by collapsing the affected lung. As a part of this procedure they were fluoroscoped (a procedure involving a continuous X-ray picture, as opposed to having a single film taken), using equipment which gave out between ten and twenty times the radiation of today's mammography equipment. Because these women were later found to have a higher than expected level of breast cancer it was said that X-rays should be kept away from breasts at all costs.

Similarly, a report came out after studying the effects of radiation on the breasts of women who survived the Hiroshima – Nagasaki atomic bombs. They too had higher levels of breast cancer than would be expected. These two reports frightened many women off having X-rays of any kind near their breasts in case the rays themselves might *produce* breast cancer. It is now known that there is no danger of this at all with modern equipment. Anyway, even if there were a provable small risk we should have to weigh it against the proven life-saving potential of the procedure. One large American study found that one-third of existing breast cancers were not able to be felt and were found only by mammography! The amount of suffering that can be prevented and the numbers of years of life that can be saved probably outweigh any possible dangers there might be.

So what is mammography used for?

1. Sorting out the cause of a breast lump.
2. Sorting out difficult thickenings felt in the breast.
3. Trying to find a cause for otherwise undiagnosable breast symptoms (nipple discharge etc).
4. Looking for disease in the opposite breast if one breast has a lump.
5. Helping surgeons plan their operations.
6. To examine very large breasts that are difficult to examine manually (lumps in these breasts can easily be missed if small or may not be detected until they're very large). Large breasts also seem to produce better X-ray pictures than do small ones and the diagnosis can be very accurate.
7. As a routine screening procedure (see page 155).
8. To put a woman's mind at rest if she fears she has cancer.

So as you can see, it's a useful, harmless, quick procedure that can yield excellent results. The best results are obtained in conjunction with a careful and skilful physical examination. Undoubtedly mammography will be further improved technically. Colour mammography is already available in some centres and computerized techniques that have proved so valuable in the body scanner will no doubt be applied to mammography in the future.

One advance on mammography is xeroradiography.

XERORADIOGRAPHY

Xerography was invented in 1937 and has since become a household process as the basis of photocopying. In 1952 the medical application of xerography (xeroradiography) started to be considered but at this time the prevailing opinion was that photographic film was, and looked likely for some time to be, a better method of capturing X-ray images. Technology has moved along quickly, though, as in other areas of medicine and science, and the process is now valuable and reliable but still not as useful as mammography.

The principle is as follows. A metallic plate is charged with electricity. This draws positive ions to the surface of the plate which is then put in a cassette just like a piece of photographic film for an X-ray. The plate is placed under the breast and X-rays are shot through the breast as with a mammogram. The X-rays alter the pattern of the electrical charge on the metallic plate and the pattern is developed using a finely particulate plastic powder. By changing the electric charge on the plate the doctor can choose to look at either a positive or negative image. The powder image is transferred to paper and heated to produce a permanent record which looks like a bluish photograph.

Xeroradiography is especially useful in examining the breasts of young women because their breasts are dense and can be difficult to visualize with ordinary mammography. This method may therefore be the choice for young women.

Two xeroradiographic views are made at right angles to each other just as with a mammogram and the procedure is, of course, totally painless. Several surveys have found the method to be as accurate as mammography and there are claims that even very small tumours can be detected. The ability to detect small tumours that haven't yet become palpable (that is, they can't be felt by doctor or patient) is an important advantage of both mammography and xeroradiography. Clinically undetectable cancers make up 43 per cent of those eventually found in women aged thirty-one to forty but only 18 per cent of those in the over-seventies. Some cancers in young women reach 6 – 8 cm (2½ – 3 inches) in diameter before they can be felt, especially if the breasts are large. Mammography and xeroradiography can often pick up these lumps while they are still easily treatable.

THERMOGRAPHY

This is a technique that measures the temperature of the skin over the breast. A doctor then relates these findings to what's going on underneath. Thermography was developed because it was found that the majority of cancers of the breast put out more heat than did the surrounding tissues. A difference of 1.5°C is not uncommon.

Essentially thermography measures infra-red radiation emitted by the skin. This is then converted directly to temperature values. The radiation can be detected either by contact thermography or telethermography. Contact thermography uses liquid cholesterol crystals that change colour under the influence of infra-red light. Tele-thermography uses optical systems to capture the infra-red light which is then converted into electrical currents and displayed on a photographic plate or a TV-type screen. Modern equipment enables the viewer to see temperature differences of 0.1°C displayed in colour very clearly and accurately.

The woman to be examined is placed in a constant-temperature room without draughts and must have her breasts exposed for at least ten minutes so that they come into balance with the room temperature. Once this temperature equilibration has taken place the actual examination itself only takes about five minutes. Most clinics take several pictures in black and white and colour.

Thermography involves no X-rays and the woman herself isn't touched as part of the procedure. It is therefore completely harmless. Unfortunately it isn't very accurate as it is now known that about a third of all breast cancers produce no heat-detectable patterns. Also the method can be 'misled' by other conditions that produce heat. A mosquito bite, sunburn, a scratch on the skin, underlying bronchitis in the chest and so on can all increase the breasts' skin temperature and give false results. It is really only useful when repeated tests are done under exactly comparable conditions in the same woman. As thermography is so safe, some centres advise that it should be used to decide who should have mammography but it is a method of breast examination that may never be widely useful, except on specific women.

Considerable research has been carried out especially in Europe into 'risk factors' or predictors of breast cancers. Thermography patterns are used in some European centres as a prognostic tool to highlight those women who should be carefully followed up using more accurate methods, but this use of thermography has not caught on elsewhere. Perhaps with increasing computerization thermography could be refined to detect underlying temperature changes but other advances are likely to overtake it. One such is ultrasound.

ULTRASOUND

This method of examining internal organs and producing pictures of them will be well known to those readers who have had a 'scan' of their baby during pregnancy. Ultrasound scanning involves the passing of high frequency sound waves into the body or an organ and then the building up of a picture from the differentially reflected waves as they bounce back off the structures inside the body. This is the same principle as is used in a marine echo sounder but it has been computerized and greatly refined for medical use.

Ultrasound is as yet very primitive in what it can offer in breast disease even though hopes were high when it was first introduced. Because it uses no radiation, can produce very good pictures (on a TV screen or on photographic film) for permanent record, and is easy to do it should have a future. It already is useful for showing up cysts which are obscured by fibrous tissue and which are thus difficult to see on mammography, but it has a long way to go before it becomes valuable for visualizing other breast lumps. At present ultrasound is complementary to other diagnostic methods but this could change.

Screening for breast cancer

While all of the methods outlined in this chapter can detect many different kinds of breast conditions, the one that doctors and their patients are really looking for is cancer. It seems logical to assume that if a cancer is caught early enough it can be cured, but this is not necessarily the case. There is a lot of conflicting research on the value of routine screening of women with no detectable breast lumps. To be effective, screening must detect the lump well before the woman would otherwise have noticed it herself.

For example, the total life expectancy of a woman aged forty-five who is felt to have an average risk of developing breast cancer is 77.7 years. The probability of her ever getting breast cancer is 6.6 per cent and the probability of her ever dying of breast cancer is 4 per cent. If this woman had a physical examination of her breasts every year but never had a mammogram her life expectancy would be increased by fifty days. Her probability of ever dying from breast cancer would be reduced from 4 per cent to 3 per cent. If this same woman were to have an annual physical examination and mammography every other year her total life expectancy could be increased by seventy-two days. So only very modest gains can be expected from screening the female population generally and screening costs a great deal of money. It is very tempting to think that by screening all women regularly breast cancer could be wiped out. Unfortunately there is little evidence that this *could* be true and anyway the costs involved are so enormous that it would be almost impossible to justify such expenditure.

Although breast cancer affects 7 per cent of women, and that is a huge number of individuals, we've seen that screening gives these women only limited benefits in terms of increased life expectancy. In view of this, the enormous expenditure involved in screening all women is not thought to be justifiable. For example, one USA survey team calculated that allowing $75 for each clinical examination, approximately $3.6 billions would be needed to examine every American woman aged thirty-five or more every year. In the UK about six million women would have to be screened to save one thousand lives a year, and that would cost £70 million – an average of £70,000 for each life.

The cost of screening is, of course, in addition to that spent on actually treating the cancers so detected. It can be argued that it is cheaper to treat early cancer picked up on screening than late cancer found only when it produces symptoms. However, the cost of screening far outweighs this slight difference.

The extra suffering caused to each individual woman whose cancer is only detected late is impossible to quantify financially. In personal if not national terms, though, this has to be considered.

As we shall see, breast cancer is the biggest cancer killer in women. One in every fourteen newborn girls will develop it and in the USA one woman dies of it every seventeen minutes. Because of these horrific statistics women naturally want to have the best possible chance of ensuring that the disease, if present, can be detected and treated as early as possible.

There are, however, risks to screening for breast cancer. First and foremost is the kindling of considerable anxiety among the population which is being screened. It is difficult, if not impossible, to put any figures on this but by constantly drawing women's attention to their potential for breast cancer it could be argued that their quality of life is being reduced even when they haven't got the disease. Secondly, the efficacy of any screening programme is dependent upon the extent to which it results in identifying disease at a stage at which it can be treated. Simply finding disease that is so far advanced that its detection becomes academic is of little value to anyone and very expensive as well.

Any screening method that produces too high a level of suspicion could easily worry millions of women unnecessarily and countless thousands of them will end up having unnecessary biopsies or even unnecessary definitive treatment. Mammography is particularly at fault here because it cannot distinguish between small malignant and small non-malignant lumps. Screening therefore means that many quite harmless lumps will be removed unnecessarily. Most experts agree that the ratio of harmless lumps to cancer lumps is about 4 or 5 to 1 but even though doctors aren't bothered by this, women certainly are. After all, every questionable lump discovered raises tremendous anxieties in the whole family and the woman is left with a scar on her breast.

Another danger of any screening programme is that of false reassurance. Many women, thinking that a particular screening programme completely rules out any possibility of cancer, assume that they are unlikely to get it and then ignore problems or tell-tale signs when they do occur. Cancer can, of course, develop between screening procedures. It has to start some time.

Another risk of screening programmes is that connected with the actual methods used. We have seen that mammography is very safe but even today with very safe machines most experts don't like to use mammography *routinely* in women under forty. This does not diminish the proven value of mammography in women with symptoms, when it is a very useful tool in assessing disease.

Of course the benefit we're all looking for from screening is that women with a breast cancer (which at the moment we can't prevent) might have their disease picked up early enough to get treatment started as soon as possible in the hopes that they might live longer. There is, sadly, no evidence that any currently used method of screening reduces absolute mortality rates from breast cancer but experts the world over are convinced that early detection of the disease improves the survival rate to some extent and almost certainly improves the quality of the woman's remaining life. For example, a small lump caught early means that less disfiguring breast surgery will be needed.

So what we all have to do, whether we are women or doctors, is to find the balance between the disadvantages and the possible benefits of breast cancer screening.

Which guidelines are reasonable to follow? It is now widely accepted that if you fall into one of the following groups you should be screened for breast cancer regularly:

1. If you have had breast cancer previously you should be screened annually no matter what your age.
2. If you have any major 'risk factors' (immediate blood relations with breast cancer, other reproductive system cancer, and a few other risk factors that are of variable importance according to which of the experts one listens to) you should be screened annually from the age of forty.
3. If you have had breast disease of any kind in the past you should be screened annually over the age of forty.
4. If you are over fifty you should be screened twice a year.

If you have ever had breast cancer you should have a physical examination carried out by a doctor and a mammogram every year. You should also examine your own breasts every month (as indeed should all women).

If your mother or sister had or has breast cancer you should be screened annually over the age of forty.

These then are the main guidelines for 'professional' screening and they can be proven to be valuable. But self-examination of the breasts should still be done monthly along the lines discussed on page 134 to detect any disease as early as possible even if you are being screened professionally. It is very difficult to be dogmatic about the absolute numbers of lives saved by self-examination because women vary very greatly in the thoroughness and regularity with which they examine themselves. However, several reports show that self-examination can reduce mortality by 18–24 per cent judged by five-year survival figures. Tumours diagnosed at self-examination do tend to be at an earlier stage in their development than those found by doctors and in those discovered accidentally by the patient. Tumours found during routine examination are usually about 20 per cent smaller than those found accidentally and this must influence the outlook to some extent.

However, one major US survey found that only 51 per cent of women practising breast self-examination did so regularly on a monthly basis and that many of them did it very badly.

So overall, for the woman who examines herself carefully and systematically every month, the chances are that she'll pick up a cancer if it is there at a stage at which it stands the best possible chance of cure and minimal disfiguring surgery. This is the best we can hope for until prevention makes inroads into the disease process itself.

CHAPTER 8

Breast cancer

When we told people we were going to write a book about the breast almost all of them said, 'Oh, it'll be all about cancer, will it?' Of course it is not, as you will have seen by now, but today's woman can be forgiven for thinking that a book about the breast would be all about cancer because the Western world has gone overboard on the subject.

The truth of the matter is as follows. Breast cancer is the commonest cancer among women, accounting for about 30 per cent of all cancers. This year approximately 25,000 women will develop the disease in the UK (110,000 in the USA) and about 14,000 will die from it (35,000 in the USA). One in every fourteen newborn girls will develop the disease and in the USA a woman will die every seventeen minutes from the disease.

Now these are amazing figures and are nothing to be complacent about, but this still means that only *7 per cent of women will get the disease*. Put another way — 93 per cent of women will never get it! So there is no need to be alarmed unnecessarily. There is, however, every need to be vigilant so that a lump, once felt, can be treated quickly and effectively. Eight out of ten lumps are *not* breast cancer and even when the diagnosis does turn out to be cancer it doesn't mean a death sentence. Six out of ten cancers grow very slowly and many women with breast cancer live long and trouble-free lives and die of something else.

Many women, especially in the USA, have become obsessed with cancer and breast cancer in particular. While it is obviously a very unpleasant disease one should bear in mind that in the same year (1979) that there were 12,091 breast cancer deaths in England and Wales, more than 9,000 women died on the roads, in accidents and through suicide and 32,400 died from 'flu and pneumonia. Before you say, 'But 'flu and pneumonia only kill old people,' just bear in mind that the majority of women dying from breast cancer are over sixty years old.

Breast cancer has become a major talking point among Western women who, encouraged by famous women who had the disease and talked about it publicly (Liz Fraser, Ingrid Bergman, Betty Ford, Shirley Temple Black, Happy Rockefeller and Anna Neagle are just some examples), are now more open on the subject than ever before. This is undoubtedly a good thing but also has the negative effect of focusing women's attention on the disease to an unnatural and unnecessary degree. Striking a balance with such an emotional and emotive subject is, however, very difficult.

No one knows how common breast cancer was in distant historical times but an accurate count of breast cancer patients was made in the USA in 1937 when ten large urban communities were surveyed. What *is* alarming about breast cancer is that in spite of all the so-called advances in both prevention and treatment the occurrence rate of breast cancer hasn't changed since this 1937 study and the outlook in terms of life expectancy once a woman has the disease hasn't changed over the last decade. There is also a suggestion that breast cancer is occurring more often among younger women since 1930 and that this may be secondary to the two-years-earlier onset of menstruation that has occurred over this time.

However, the overall incidence of breast cancer hasn't *increased* either since the 1930s: the medical and health lobbies are simply shouting about it a lot more to try to get women to look for and report their breast lumps early so that they stand a better chance of a cure. To some extent this campaign of fear, which has often been exaggerated, is justifiable but on the reverse of the coin are those women who now equate every breast lump with cancer and every cancer with imminent death. Neither of these fears is grounded in truth, as we shall see.

The fact that the occurrence rate of breast cancer hasn't changed is depressing from everyone's point of view, especially in light of the fact that so much money and human endeavour have been poured into research in this field. But there's good news too because, if the rate of breast cancer is still the same, today's woman is no *more* likely to get it than her mother was and it's still a fact that 93 per cent of women will never get it. Only twenty-two per 100,000 women aged thirty and over will develop a breast cancer in any one year but this rises to 301 per 100,000 at the age of eighty.

None of this, however, takes away from the fact that thousands of women *do* die every year in the Western world from breast cancer and that countless thousands more are put to inconvenience, are hospitalized, are subjected to emotional turmoil, suffer the side effects of various treatments or are even mutilated by surgery. Clearly anything that can be done to relieve the incidence of the disease would be welcomed with open arms so let's look at some of the theories and what, if anything, can be done to prevent breast cancer occurring in the first place.

The causes

First of all let's get one thing clear. There is no single cause of breast cancer. On the contrary, it is highly likely that it is caused by several factors. We saw in Chapter 1 that the way in which a modern woman's breasts function throughout her reproductive life is very different from that for which they were designed, and we feel that this very recent and totally unsound (in biological terms) behaviour is at the root of many breast conditions, cancer included. So given that reproductive experience seems to be so important, let's start there.

Reproductive experience seems to play an important part in the incidence of breast cancer. A recent collaborative study in seven culturally very different centres around the world found that the risk of breast cancer is related to the age at which a woman bears her first full-term child. Women who have their first baby before the age of eighteen have about one-third of the risk of getting breast cancer compared with those who put off their first baby until thirty-five or more. To be protective at all, it seems that the first pregnancy must occur before thirty – indeed, women having their first babies after the age of thirty have a higher risk of breast cancer than those who never have babies, and studies of nuns and other non-childbearing women show that the risk in such women is already very high.

It also seems that the protective effect of childbearing is limited to the first birth. Other babies, even at an early age, seem to confer little additional protection. It's also interesting that such protection only occurs as the result of a full-term pregnancy. Where the link between abortion (miscarriage) and breast cancer has been studied it has been found to increase the incidence of the cancer and not decrease it.

So, as one would expect from what we said in Chapter 1, a pregnancy within a few years of the onset of menstruation seems to protect a woman from breast cancer. The fact that the reduction in incidence is so great suggests that this early reproductive phase in a woman's life is one during which tumour cells can form and start to grow. It has been suggested that the first pregnancy acts as a kind of trigger effect which either permanently alters the factors responsible for 'high risk' or otherwise so alters the breast that it is less likely to undergo malignant change. The older a woman is when she has her first pregnancy, the more likely she is to have a tumour or potential tumour cells in her breasts at the time of the pregnancy.

Breastfeeding has been thought for about fifty years now to reduce the likelihood of breast cancer in the woman who breastfeeds but argument still rages on the subject. Various studies, notably in Japan (a low-risk area for breast cancer), have shown that lactation is protective. One piece of research is worth commenting on. It was conducted with the help of the boat women of Aberdeen, Hong Kong. By cultural tradition these women feed their infants from their right breasts only. More than 90 per cent of those over thirty-five practise this custom but the younger ones are abandoning it. One possible reason for the custom is that the traditional Chinese dress buttons up on the right side so making the right breast more accessible than the left. The research team found that in thirty-four women with cancers who had breast-fed, twenty-three cancers occurred in the left and eleven in the right breast, a ratio of 2:1. In women over fifty-five with breast cancer the ratio was 3:1 in favour of the left breast. In non-boat women in the same area the ratio of left to right was 1:1.

This and other studies suggested that breastfeeding somehow protected the breasts from cancer but recent worldwide studies do not bear this out. A recent study in Tokyo among women with more than five years' (and some with more than ten years') lactation experience found that breast cancers were just as common among them as among control patients.

But we have to take issue with the world cancer experts on this because it is very unlikely that the vast majority of women who are 'breastfeeding' their babies are doing so in the way that the hunter-gatherers did in the past. Most women's ideas of breastfeeding (except in very traditional, rural parts of the world) are conditioned by our modern, Western approach, which involves very little nipple stimulation and correspondingly low prolactin levels being produced by the pituitary gland.

The !Kung that we discussed in Chapter 1 breastfeed their young very frequently but briefly (with only thirteen minutes between feeds on average). This produces consistently very high prolactin levels instead of the occasional peaks of the hormone seen in most of today's women who, even if they are 'enlightened', may only feed every hour or so and then hardly at all during the night because their baby sleeps in another room. Studies of the !Kung and other tribes have shown that a baby left lying next to his mother feeds spontaneously (often without waking the mother) about every ten to fifteen minutes during the night. There really can be no comparison between this type of breastfeeding and the continuously high prolactin levels it produces and most people's ideas of breastfeeding today, so data based on women who have 'breast-fed' may be useless unless they have fed in this way. To say that the kind of token breastfeeding (albeit over several years) that is currently practised around the world today does not protect against breast cancer is almost certainly true. Where so many (even expert) people go astray when talking of the protective nature of breastfeeding against various conditions is that they concentrate on the baby at the breast and the nutrition he is getting. In hunter-gatherers (and indeed in any woman who breastfeeds on a completely unrestricted basis) babies are often at the breast simply for comfort a lot of the time. This 'comfort sucking' as it is called, nevertheless results in prolonged and frequent periods of nipple stimulation which in turn has profound hormonal effects on the mother. And don't forget that historically such high hormone levels were the norm because most women were pregnant or breastfeeding for most of their reproductive lives. In this state of affairs the woman rarely ovulated as we saw in Chapter 1. This leads naturally to the next factor in the development of breast cancer.

The ovaries seem to play an interesting, if not vital, role in the causation of breast cancer. The best evidence for an ovarian role in the disease is the finding that levels of breast cancer in women who have had their ovaries removed surgically are lower than would be expected. The effect seems to be greater the younger the woman is when her ovaries are removed. Most recent studies have found that there is a 40 per cent reduction in breast cancer risk after the operation with the best results if the woman was under thirty-five at the time of the procedure. Even thirty years later the breast cancer risk among women whose ovaries had been removed before the age of forty-five is only about half that for women who had experienced a natural menopause. More than a quarter of women in the USA have their ovaries removed but the number having the operation at an age young enough to influence the development of breast cancer is small. This is why the overall incidence of breast cancer is very little reduced by this common operation.

We saw in Chapter 1 that our ancient ancestors started menstruating later and had an earlier menopause, so reducing their effective reproductive life-span. Recent research has followed this up with breast cancer in mind. Studies have shown that women who start to menstruate young have a greater risk of developing breast cancer compared with controls. A Polish study, for example, found that women who had their first period before sixteen had 1.8 times the risk of developing breast cancer as those who started later. Other studies show that a late natural menopause is also associated with an increased breast cancer risk and that women who have a natural menopause at fifty-five or over have twice the risk of women who stop menstruating before the age of forty-five.

All of this fits very well with the changing profile of today's female reproductive lifestyle and the considerable increase in breast cancer that has occurred over the centuries as women's reproductive life-spans have increased.

There seems to be considerable *international variation* in the incidence of breast cancer and this has proved an interesting, if fairly unfruitful, area of research in the subject. Rates are five to six times more common in North America and northern Europe compared with Asia and Africa. Southern European and South American women have breast cancer rates somewhere between the two. Where rates are high, the risk increases through life and where rates are low, the risk increases with age until middle life, then reaches a plateau and, after about the age of fifty, declines. No one can explain this.

Genetics is an obvious place to start but no evidence seems to back up such a theory. On the contrary, the breast cancer rates of immigrant women tend to mirror those of the host country, pointing to the possibility that breast cancer might be an environmental disease (see below). Many women reading this will immediately assume that the low breast cancer rates in Africa and Asia probably have something to do with the way in which Asian and African women run their reproductive lives and there may indeed be something in this argument. Unfortunately it's not that simple. Twenty-nine per cent of a sample of general hospital patients in Sao Paulo, Brazil had had their first baby before the age of twenty, and 81 per cent by thirty; in

Boston, USA, the figures were 8 per cent and 58 per cent respectively. Other knowledge of cancer rates suggests that on these figures the breast cancer rates in Boston should have been 30 per cent higher than in Sao Paulo but in fact they were twice as high! Even climatic temperature has been looked at to try to explain the international differences in breast cancer rates but nothing has come out of this approach.

Diet certainly could be a factor in explaining the international differences in the disease. Human breast cancers are often hormone-dependent tumours and dietary influences are known to affect the production and action of various hormones in the body. But the food we eat is enormously complex and there are many possible ways in which it could make women prone to breast cancer.

It has been known for some years that women who are obese are more prone to breast cancer. A study in Taiwan found that women weighing more than 55 kg (just over 8½ stone) had a breast cancer risk twice that of those weighing less than 45 kg (just over 7 stone) and that the risk was greater among women over fifty than among younger women. Recent research has found that fatty tissue produces a type of oestrogen as a metabolic waste-product and this has led researchers to question the possibility that it is these non-ovarian oestrogens that are 'feeding' the tumour cells in the breast.

Dietary intake has been positively correlated with breast cancer in several studies. People on high-fat diets have higher proportions of certain bacteria in their bowels. These bacteria are able to produce oestrogens from the increased level of biliary steroids the high-fat diet also produces. Such oestrogens are known to be potentially carcinogenic to the breast.

Other interesting research is pointing to the implication of milk and dairy products. This research began when it was noticed that there was a relationship between the prevalence of lactase deficiency − a condition in which the intestine contains insufficient lactase to split up milk sugar (lactose) effectively − and breast cancer. Lactase, the intestinal enzyme that splits the milk sugar lactose, is present in the intestines of all mammals immediately after birth. After weaning, however, lactase production usually falls off and in most adult mammals there is none: they are incapable of digesting lactose. Most human populations follow the same pattern with low levels of lactase in their intestines and almost no intake of milk as adults. The exceptions to this rule are the peoples living in the few countries in which there is a tradition of dairying. They have high levels of lactase in their intestines. In these populations milk and other dairy product intake is high during and after childhood and breast cancer rates are high too.

Several international studies have linked mortality from breast cancer to the intake of cows' milk and even the consumption of other dairy products (cheese and butter in particular) is so linked. So what could this link be between milk, other dairy products and breast cancer?

The answer is that no one knows for sure but there are several theories — each with good research to back it up. Perhaps they are even all interrelated in some way. Certainly when one consumes a lot of milk and dairy products one consumes a lot of fat and we have seen that fat intake has been linked to breast cancer. In addition to the production of oestrogens by the body's fat stores and the production of oestrogens in the intestines (which we have already mentioned), a high fat intake and its resulting obesity lowers the age at which a girl starts menstruating (and we have seen that this is important) and also alters blood hormone levels in a way which favours the development of breast cancer. So a high-fat diet has a lot to answer for.

We have seen already that the bacterial population of the bowel is altered by a high-fat diet and milk-rich diets certainly seem to do this too. It is possible, though not proven, that milk encourages the growth of bacteria that produce carcinogenic oestrogens in the bowel.

But it's not just the fat content of cows' milk that might be the culprit. There are large numbers of other biologically active substances in cows' milk that might be responsible for breast cancer. Human breast tissue is influenced by many different hormones and even plant oestrogens have been found to be biologically active in human breast cancer cells in laboratory experiments, markedly increasing tumour cell proliferation. Plant oestrogens and many other hormones are known to be present in cows' milk but not enough is yet known about the amounts entering human blood from the intestines, or about their actions.

Murine (mouse) milk contains a tumour-producing virus which causes breast cancer in mice and very similar particles have been found in human milk, although the significance of them is not known. It's possible that cows' milk contains similar virus particles and that they could be a factor in human breast cancer.

Several hormonal substances have been used as growth-promoters in cattle including various female sex hormones. Antibiotics, pesticides and many other substances also find their way into cows' milk and may be significant in humans if they are subjected to large enough quantities for long enough. We simply don't know.

What we can say though is that cows' milk is a food for the nourishment of calves. There is no reason to believe that it is ideally suitable for human nutrition and there is increasing evidence that it is not the wholesome, unobnoxious food we have all been brainwashed into thinking it is. We are the only animal species that regularly consumes the milk meant for the young of another species and we are almost certainly paying the price for it.

Another dietary change that links our high-fat diet to breast-cancer is our increasing consumption of highly refined foods and hand in hand with this our falling consumption of dietary fibre. There is now an enormous body of research from all over the world on the subject of dietary fibre and there is no doubt that people who eat lots of fibre (roughage) have substantially different bacterial populations in their bowels compared with those who eat a highly refined diet. Although, as far as we are aware, no studies have been done linking breast cancer with dietary fibre intake, it cannot escape one's notice that people in those countries in which breast cancer is so common consume very little fibre. Current theories point to a low-fibre diet as being a key factor in the production of bowel cancer (the second biggest cancer killer in the Western world). Conversely, a high-fibre diet may be protective against both bowel and breast cancers because of the way it alters intestinal bacteria in favour of 'safer' bacterial growth. Such a diet may well also have a beneficial side effect on the oestrogen production from the biliary steroids we mentioned above. So in summary, a high-fat, low-fibre diet has a key role to play in the production of bowel cancer. There is good cause to question whether the same mechanisms might not also produce excessive amounts of carcinogenic oestrogens that then act on the breast.

In conclusion then, overnutrition, the consumption of too much fat and milk and the very low levels of dietary fibre seen in countries in which breast cancer rates are so high could well be risk factors for the disease. Recent research in California, since repeated around the world, has shown that a low-fat diet, rich in unrefined carbohydrate, is very much more healthy in all kinds of provable ways. It is close to what our hunter-gatherer ancestors ate and we haven't been around long enough yet to be able to ignore their behaviour – our bodies are still biologically the same as theirs. We saw in Chapter 1 that we have revolutionized our reproductive behaviour, possibly to our cost. It is now apparent that we have similarly altered our eating habits. The results of this may be equally unacceptable.

The higher levels of breast cancer among *families* has long been known. Female relatives of women with breast cancer have two to three times the general population's breast cancer rate. One survey reported that breast cancer shows 'anticipation', with daughters of affected women experiencing the disease younger than did their mothers. Relatives of women with bilateral breast cancer (cancer affecting both breasts) have three times the risk of relatives of women with a single breast involved. This means that female relatives of a woman with bilateral cancer have a 45 per cent chance of developing the cancer in their lifetime.

Other cancers found in association with breast cancer have also given food for thought and provoked much research. A recent study, for example, found that between 7 and 10 per cent of women with breast cancer eventually developed a tumour in the other breast – a tumour which is a second primary and *not* a secondary tumour which had spread from the first one. This emphasizes the importance of following up women who have had one tumour diagnosed. Nearly 10 per cent will have another. The same biological conditions that produced the first one are still there, after all.

Cancer of the breast is also associated with an increased risk of tumours in certain other sites. Tumours of the endometrium (the lining of the uterus) occur much more frequently in those women who have a breast cancer (and the converse is true) than would be expected and women who have cancer of the body of the uterus (not the cervix) have a rate of breast cancer 1.3 – 2.0 times greater than the normal. The association of breast cancer and cancer of the ovary is not well established but some studies have found a link.

Cancer of the colon is associated with a higher than expected level of breast cancer and one survey found that women with breast cancer or endometrial cancer had about twice the expected risk of having a cancer of the colon. We have seen that both breast and colon cancer are associated with a high fat intake and it is possible that they are also associated with a low dietary fibre intake too. These two dietary abnormalities go hand in hand in almost every population studied around the world. It is possible then that our strange diet produces carcinogens for the colon (acting locally) and the breast (acting via the bloodstream).

Viruses have long been a favourite of the 'causes of cancer' brigade and as long ago as 1936 mouse breast cancer was linked to the presence of a cancer factor which today we know to be a virus particle. Interest in the possibility that human breast cancer might be caused by a virus was re-kindled by reports that there were virus particles in human milk similar to the cancer-producing ones found in mice. However, in spite of the smoke, no fire has yet been discovered. Even if a virus is responsible its mode of transmission is somewhat dubious. There is no evidence that women who were themselves breast-fed have an increased risk of developing the disease. On the contrary, in countries where breastfeeding rates are low, cancer rates are high, and conversely. A viral cause for human breast cancer is still not proven – if indeed there is one to prove.

Oestrogens seem to play a vital role in the production and growth of some breast cancers. We have already looked at the evidence surrounding ovarian function and its connection with breast cancer. All women produce oestrogens, yet only 7 per cent will develop a breast cancer, so clearly there is no simple cause-and-effect mechanism at work. As we pointed out in Chapter 1, we believe the answer will probably lie in the large number of menstrual cycles modern women experience, cycles which send hundreds of surges of oestrogens around the body instead of the twenty to thirty our hunter-gatherer ancestors would have experienced.

Other ideas about the role of oestrogens arise from the fact that women produce three different types of these hormones. Two of these (oestrone and oestradiol) readily produce breast cancers in rats and mice but the third (oestriol) does not. Studies have suggested that women with a low ratio of oestriol to the other fractions have a high cancer risk but evidence is conflicting as yet. Women from different areas around the world have different ratios of these three types of oestrogen in their urine (and hence in their blood) and it is possible that further studies of this will provide the answers we're looking for.

Oestrogens taken in the form of the contraceptive Pill seem to have no effect on breast cancer one way or the other (except by delaying the first pregnancy so easily). Certainly they do not protect against breast cancer as they do against benign (non-cancerous) breast disease.

The discovery of hormone receptors in breast tissue has further increased our knowledge and understanding of the role of oestrogens in some breast cancers. This subject is discussed in more detail on page 197.

Prolactin is a hormone produced by the pituitary gland. Its levels are increased during pregnancy and in response to nipple stimulation, increasing two- to twenty-fold in the blood during five to fifteen minutes of mechanical stimulation of the nipple. This rise in prolactin levels occurs in all women whether they are lactating or not. Breast-feeding women produce extremely high levels of prolactin in their blood, the purpose of which is only partly known. Perhaps besides producing milk, high prolactin levels are linked to the suppression of ovulation that occurs during breastfeeding but this is still not clear.

At the moment the interaction between prolactin and oestrogens in the initiation of or the growth of breast cancer is entirely speculative but research currently under way will undoubtedly produce some answers soon. It seems that the more pregnancies a woman has and possibly the longer she breastfeeds on an unrestricted basis, the greater is her protection from breast cancer (especially if her first pregnancy is under the age of twenty) so perhaps prolactin (which is only normally produced in really large amounts during pregnancy and lactation) could be protective against breast cancer in some way.

Recent research in the USA suggests that women who use *barrier contraceptives* are more likely to suffer from breast cancer than are other women. No one knows why this should be but it is quite possible that something in a man's semen acts in the woman to protect her from developing the cancer. It has been postulated that the immune system of a woman using barrier contraception may be unprepared to cope with cancerous changes and that her breast cells are thus put at a greater risk, but there is as yet no evidence on this. It's certainly an exciting observation, especially as barrier methods (notably the sheath) are the most commonly used form of artificial contraceptive in the West.

Ionizing radiation has long been thought to be a cause of breast cancer. This is discussed on page 151 when considering the safety of mammography.

So, in summary, it can be seen that no one yet knows what causes breast cancer and the chances are that it will turn out to be caused by several interlinked factors. There *is* enough known, though, to be able to draw up a profile of the woman who is least likely to suffer from the disease. She'll be of normal or slightly below normal weight as a child (so that her periods will start later); she'll have her first child under the age of twenty; she will breastfeed each child for at least a year or two on an unrestricted basis; she'll go on the Pill between babies (of which she'll have at least three or four) and otherwise use the natural birth spacing provided by prolonged and unrestricted breastfeeding until she is sterilized after her last baby; she'll eat a healthy diet rich in dietary fibre and low in dairy foods and fat; and she will avoid becoming overweight.

There's little most of us can do about many of the risk factors for breast cancer but there is no doubt that by adhering to this plan we could dramatically reduce a woman's chances of getting breast cancer. Understandably very few women are likely to be willing to adopt such a lifestyle and so will continue to expose themselves to an increased risk of developing the disease.

The symptoms of breast cancer

The main symptom of breast cancer is a lump. Over 90 per cent of those with a breast cancer complain first of a lump. It is usually hard, in one breast only, irregular in shape, with a poorly defined outline, immobile, painless and non-tender. Most cancers occur in the upper, outer quadrant of the breast.

But cancer can produce other symptoms. Pain occurs in about one in ten women but nipple discharge is the most common symptom after a lump. The discharge that is typical of an underlying cancer comes from one nipple duct, arises spontaneously and is straw-coloured, or straw-coloured tinged with blood. Rarely it is watery. Sometimes retraction (a pulling in) or elevation of the nipple is the first sign or there may be eczema on the nipple skin.

Skin symptoms such as dimpling, orange peel skin (see page 140), redness, or even ulceration can be the first sign. Rarely women complain of lumps in their armpits or pains in other parts of the body (produced by distant spread of the tumour).

What to do if you find a lump

The simple answer is 'go to your doctor straight away'. Tell him what you've found and he'll examine you. If you're not at ease going to your own general practioner, go to a Well-Woman clinic or even to a family planning clinic. Whatever you do don't delay because we now know that delay has a price in unnecessary suffering and even possibly in lives.

Quite often a woman goes to her doctor only to be told that the lump is one of the many 'normal' ones that can occur or to be reassured that it doesn't feel at all like a cancer. The odds are greatly in favour (four to one) of the lump being non-cancerous, so don't get alarmed unnecessarily. For more details of what a doctor will do to make the diagnosis see page 147.

The treatment of breast cancer: what can be done?

The natural development of breast cancers is that some grow rapidly and others slowly. About six out of ten are slow growers and of the four out of ten that are fast growers, nearly all will have caused death within six years of their discovery. Some will already have spread to bones around the body by the time they are first discovered and some will remain contained within the breast for a long time. Survival rates for *untreated* breast cancer are depressing. Only about a fifth of such women live for as long as five years, although some live much longer. With the best treatment of the earliest cancers, three-quarters of affected women are alive five years later and about a half ten years after the diagnosis is made. So it's well worth getting help.

As with so many conditions in which there is no single cure-all technique, the field of breast cancer is a battleground for the exponents of many, varied treatments. There are no hard and fast rules and if one were to listen to twenty top breast cancer specialists discussing how they would want their wives' cancers managed (if these cancers were similar in type and stage), they'd all have an individual viewpoint. Basically, the way that breast cancer is managed depends to some degree on the stage it has reached by the time the diagnosis is made. The staging of breast cancers is a complex subject but there are generally considered to be four stages. It can be useful to know what stage any given tumour is at because it can influence the treatment that is chosen.

Stage 1 tumours are less than 5 cm (2 inches) in diameter, are not attached to the skin or to muscle and are not associated with enlarged lymph glands (nodes) in the armpit.

In stage 2 cancers, the lump is about the same size as Stage 1 but the nodes in the armpit are swollen. This indicates that the body's immune defences (many of them centred in these nodes) are being mobilized to try to kill the cancer. Such enlarged nodes contain tumour cells.

By stage 3, cancer cells have spread around the body but there are no tumours elsewhere (other than in the breast). The lump is larger than 5 cm (2 inches) across and is attached to the chest wall, to muscle or to the skin. The armpit nodes are enlarged.

Stage 4 cancer has spread to other parts of the body so the size of the breast lump or the nodes under the arm is immaterial. The size of the lump at this stage is also no indication of the seriousness of the condition.

To some extent a knowledge of the stage a cancer is at when it is discovered enables the doctor to foretell the progress of the disease — but this is by no means cut and dried.

In essence the aim in the treatment of breast cancer is primarily to control the local growth of the disease (usually by removing it). Once this has been done, or if the disease has already spread outside the breast, other therapeutic measures will have to be taken.

In order to see if and where the tumour has spread the doctor will first examine the breast thoroughly. He'll then usually take a biopsy specimen to ensure that it definitely *is* a cancer. This will be done in one of the ways outlined on page 148. In some medical centres he'll order a mammogram (a soft tissue X-ray of the breast — see page 150), a chest X-ray and a series of X-rays of the skeleton to look for secondary deposits in bones. This latter may well be done in parallel with a radioactive bone scan or liver scan to look for secondary deposits in these organs. In most hospitals not involved in research most women will not have all (or indeed many) of these tests. The surgical team then decides upon the course of treatment to follow, taking each woman as an individual case.

Very simply, a cancer confined to the breast has a 90 per cent chance of complete cure but one that has spread to the lymph nodes has only a 50 per cent chance of a cure. One that has spread to involve the bones and other organs can't be cured by surgery alone but radiotherapy and other treatments will help (see pages 194 -198).

Before we look at each of the types of treatment and what they are here is a résumé of the general principles involved in treating cancer of the breast.

CANCER CONFINED TO THE BREAST AND LOCAL LYMPH NODES
Early breast cancer is treatable with surgery alone or surgery in combination with radiotherapy and/or anti-cancer drugs. For many years now experts have disagreed about the extent of surgery necessary for cancer of the breast. It is now generally agreed that radical (that is, major) operations (see page 179) on the breast involving the removal of the whole breast together with the underlying muscle and the lymph nodes under the armpit, disfigure the woman badly yet produce no improvement in survival rates when compared with simpler operations.

Because of this, today's surgeon does not recommend it. This change of practice is having a positive side-effect on women who, previously scared about being disfigured, now come to their doctors earlier and can be treated more easily.

However, a crucial part of the treatment is still to get good local control of the disease. Because breast cancer can cause unpleasant ulcers if left untreated, it is most important to treat the primary lump adequately. For this reason many surgeons feel the best operation is to remove all the breast tissue on the affected side at an operation (see page 178) known as a simple mastectomy.

A new operation is coming on the scene and has obvious attractions. It is called a *subcutaneous mastectomy* (see page 179). In this procedure all the breast tissue is removed with the cancer cells inside yet leaving the skin of the breast intact. A silicone bag is sometimes implanted at the same operation and the woman comes round after the operation with a new normal-looking breast. Some surgeons remove only the lump and its surrounding tissue — lumpectomy (see page 178), in which case an implant is not used.

Other methods of controlling the disease locally include radiotherapy alone (see page 195) and removal of the lump in addition to radiotherapy. Although a cure is more important than worrying too much about one's figure it's encouraging to know that more surgeons today are trying to reduce the psychological insult to the woman with breast cancer who has lost a breast. Unfortunately, the successful treatment of most cancers (even early ones) involves removing the breast.

Even if the breast can't be preserved, simply removing it and possibly taking out any affected nodes under the armpit is all that is required for early cancer. Subsequent treatment depends greatly on the centre you're at. Some give radiotherapy and others reserve it until and if further trouble occurs. If radiotherapy is advised, it is not urgent but is usually started within a few weeks.

Most experts now agree that the term 'early breast cancer' may be a misnomer because the latest research suggests that even when the growth appears to be confined to the breast, it has often already spread throughout the body. If, as is now thought to be the case, breast cancer has often already spread by the time a lump is felt, the way we currently manage breast cancer will have to be re-thought and perhaps many more lumps given the full treatment regardless of their initial size. It is better to have a small lump removed rather than a big one and it has been shown that women who have small tumours removed live longer than those who have large tumours removed. The dilemmas and confusion surrounding the management of breast cancer are such that it is almost impossible to be sure what to do for the best.

CANCER THAT HAS SPREAD OUTSIDE THE BREAST

Once a breast cancer has spread to involve the rest of the body, the management of the whole condition is carried out in this light. The lump in the breast may simply be removed to prevent it ulcerating through the skin and this may be combined with radiotherapy. Often, the simplest of operations is done for the most severe form of disease as the surgeon won't want to subject the woman to unnecessary major surgery. Radiotherapy may also be used to treat secondary cancer deposits in bones so as to reduce the bone pain, which it does very effectively.

As some breast cancers seem to be influenced by a woman's hormones, various kinds of hormonal manipulations have been tried as forms of therapy. This type of treatment has been given a new lease of life with the discovery of oestrogen receptors in breast tissue. The presence or absence of these can now help doctors decide whether or not to use hormone therapies at all. For more on this, see page 197.

Women who are pre-menopausal or within five years of the

menopause can have both ovaries removed. About one-third will have breast cancers that respond to this measure within three months of the operation. At the first sign of a recurrence these women can have their adrenal glands removed, which again seems to buy more time. As a last resort, the pituitary gland can be removed, thus removing the last hormone-producing gland that could affect the growth and spread of a hormone-dependent tumour. The last two operations are less common now as anti-cancer drugs are improving. Anyway, such operations are only indicated at all if the tumour is hormone-dependent — a fact which can be ascertained by measuring oestrogen receptor levels in a piece of cancer tissue removed at a biopsy.

In those women known to have a hormone-sensitive tumour yet who don't respond to the original ovary removal, male hormones can be tried and women who are too ill to have their adrenal glands removed at an operation can have them suppressed by a drug called dexamethasone.

Anti-cancer drugs (see also page 195) have a place in the treatment of advanced breast cancer but they are often only prescribed as a last resort after other things have failed. Several drugs are often used in combination and the treatment may last for months. In pre-menopausal women, but not in post-menopausal ones, anti-cancer drugs have been shown to lengthen the disease-free interval after mastectomy in some trials but not in others.

Let's look now in more detail at the specific treatments: surgery; radiotherapy; chemotherapy (anti-cancer drugs); hormone therapy; and immunotherapy.

Surgery

Surgery for breast cancer is done for two distinct reasons. First and most commonly, it is performed to remove the lump (with or without other tissues) so as to control the growth of the local disease. Second, it is done to remove endocrine (hormone-producing) glands in an effort to control the spread and distant effects of the disease. This second indication is very much less common than the first and has already been discussed briefly on page 176.

There are six types of operation done for breast cancer but one (a simple mastectomy) is used in eight out of ten women in the UK. We'll consider each briefly in turn, starting with the simplest.

A *lumpectomy* is a lay term, now adopted by the medical profession, for a simple operation, carried out under general anaesthesia, to remove a lump alone. It is often followed by radiotherapy. Clearly, such a procedure often involves the removal of very little breast tissue if the lump is small and this is pleasant for the woman, but experts disagree as to how useful it is as a procedure for eradicating the disease. The dividing line between this procedure and a partial mastectomy is only one of degree as we shall see in the paragraph below describing the operation.

A *simple mastectomy* is an operation in which the entire breast is removed down to, but not including, the underlying chest muscles. Because the chest muscles are left intact the woman doesn't have the unpleasant disfiguring hollowness of the chest that radical mastectomy produces. Eight out of ten women in Britain with breast cancer have this type of mastectomy today and almost half of them will have the nodes under the armpit removed at the same time. In the other half, the lymph nodes under the collarbone, in the armpit and around the breast are left intact even though they may be involved in the disease.

Some surgeons also use this type of operation in women who are thought to be too poor a surgical risk for the more serious procedures. This means that a simple mastectomy is done in the elderly woman or in those whose cancer has already spread and in whom more serious breast surgery would produce little additional benefit. The operation prevents the lump from ulcerating through the skin, as it might if the operation were not done, and reduces the amount of cancer tissue present for drug or irradiation therapy to act on. Many surgeons find that a simple mastectomy combined with post-operative irradiation produces just as good a cure rate as more extensive operations. This is why simple mastectomy is now the most common operation for breast cancer.

Partial mastectomy is the name used for a procedure in which the area of the breast containing the tumour is widely excised together with a diamond-shaped section of fat tissue and skin. It is like a more extensive lumpectomy. After such an excision, the surgeon tries to re-form the breast to make it look as normal as possible but this can be difficult because about a quarter of the breast may have to be removed (more in women with large breasts). Fewer than 10 per cent of women have this type of operation.

Such a procedure is used if the cancer is still confined to the limits of the breast. Unfortunately, although it's tempting to do such an operation because women prefer less invasive surgery, evidence shows that six out of ten breast cancers have spread to other parts of the breast by the time they are operated on and that these other deposits can still kill the woman. This is another reason for the popularity of the simple mastectomy.

A *radical mastectomy* is the most extensive operation that is commonly performed today. It is still widely considered to be the best treatment for the removal of a breast cancer but is less popular with women than it is with their surgeons. 'Radical' means 'thorough' or 'complete' and this is what the operation is.

With this procedure the surgeon removes the breast itself, the underlying chest wall muscles and many of the lymph nodes in the area. The nodes are removed because it is to them that the cancer first spreads outside the breast. Unfortunately, the removal of these nodes interferes with the lymph drainage of the arm on that side which can lead to post-operative swelling of the arm. We shall see how to overcome this below. The skin all round the breast area is undermined so that it can be pulled together to cover the gap left where the breast itself was removed. If the skin can't be pulled together a skin graft from the woman's thigh can be used.

The operation is carried out under a general anaesthetic and takes about two hours.

An *extended radical mastectomy* is an even more invasive operation but is rarely done today.

A *subcutaneous mastectomy* is an operation at which the lump is removed along with the rest of the breast tissue as it is 'shelled out' of the breast skin. An implant is then inserted under the skin either during that or at a later operation to reform the contour of the breast.

Although this brief listing of the operations may seem pretty clear-cut it is not. There are almost as many opinions about breast surgery for cancer as there are surgeons and the choice of the procedure in any one woman depends very much on the individual surgeon and his experience of what works best.

The tendency today is for surgeons to do much less extensive an operation than was the case even ten years ago. This has come about because many trials have shown that radical operations simply don't increase the woman's life expectancy yet disfigure her more and produce more post-operative problems. In 1969 one in five breast cancer patients in the UK had a radical mastectomy; by 1977 the figure was only one in sixteen.

Before you have a mastectomy you owe it to yourself to discuss the whole thing with your surgeon. If you aren't happy or you think he's suggesting an approach which seems too drastic to you, say so or even seek a second opinion. Remember that there are few absolute 'rights' and 'wrongs' when it comes to breast cancer surgery and opinions vary enormously.

AFTER THE OPERATION

Coming round from the anaesthetic after having a breast off is bound to be unpleasant, especially if you went into the operation for a biopsy and frozen section (see page 149) and didn't know whether the breast would be removed. But even if you have had time to prepare yourself it's still a shock to find you're flat on one side of your chest. It's also pretty painful immediately post-operatively because the area operated

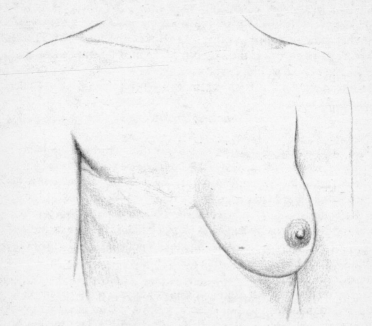

The chest wall after a mastectomy.

on is very wide and there are lots of stitches. Always ask for plenty of painkillers well in advance of needing them because otherwise you could be in pain for some hours if the staff are busy. You'll probably feel weepy but don't bottle it up. Losing a breast is a terrible blow to most women, especially in the first few days. Some women complain of pins and needles or darting sensations across their chest after the operation but these pass quickly.

Recovery after a mastectomy has three main goals: maintenance of shoulder function on the operated side; emotional adjustment; and restoration of the external appearance.

The average woman at this stage has feelings which are a mixture of disappointment, depression, anxiety, anger and relief that she's free from her cancer. At this time she needs masses of reassurance and the help of someone who has had a breast removed can be extremely valuable. Quite naturally a woman in this fragile physical and emotional state doesn't behave normally, even by her own standards, and easily finds fault with the hospital staff or simply bursts into tears at the slightest provocation. Ideally, the post-operative care of mastectomy patients should be the responsibility of a co-ordinated team including an informed and interested nurse, someone who knows about prostheses, a member of a self-help group and a physiotherapist, but this is uncommon in the UK.

PHYSICAL RECOVERY FROM BREAST SURGERY

This starts the minute you wake up and is, like the recovery from any other operation, greatly coloured by your mental attitude. As we have seen above, women who have just had a breast removed are likely to be adversely affected emotionally.

Once the first day is over, the physical pain will begin to ease and you'll be allowed out of bed. The nurse will dress the wound from time to time and you may have a drain coming through the skin to allow tissue fluid and blood to escape from the wound. This will be removed by the nurse after a few days. When the nurses are dressing your wound don't be alarmed by the appearance of the chest. Many women become very distressed, as they don't realize that all large wounds look rather unpleasant early on and that within a couple of weeks the whole area will begin to look quite reasonable again. The stitches will be taken out by the nurse after about ten days.

Although losing a breast is pretty awful, you'll be spared many of

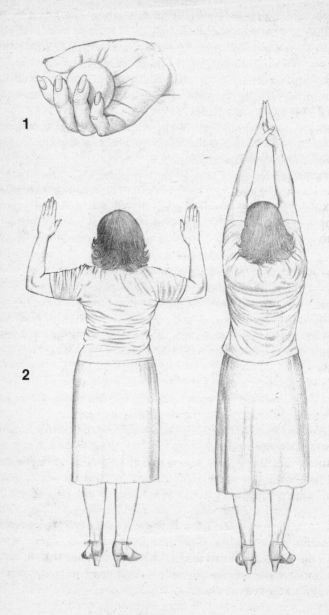

Exercises 1 and 2.

the unpleasant experiences lots of other post-operative patients have. The catheters into the bladder, the drips in the arm, the tubes into the throat and so on are not for you. You'll be able to be up and about and able to eat and drink as normal almost at once.

After a radical mastectomy you'll find it can be quite difficult to raise the arm on the operated side. This is because one of the muscles removed at the operation was attached to the arm. Even though it's awkward and painful most surgeons have found from experience that early mobilization of the arm really helps speed recovery. In some hospitals a physiotherapist will teach you what to do but if she doesn't, here's a guide.

From the second day after the operation try to do these exercises at least six times a day spread throughout the waking day. Any exercises that improve hand and shoulder movement and increase arm muscle strength will do perfectly well but here are a few suggestions.

Exercise 1: Ball exercise. Get a small soft rubber ball and squeeze it repeatedly with the hand on your affected side. It's a good idea to do this lying down with your arm elevated. This promotes drainage of the lymphatic channels and helps prevent swelling of the arm. Repeat this exercise several times a day for as long as you have any arm or hand swelling. Later, as things improve, you can sit at a sofa with your arm along the arm of the sofa to do your squeezing.

Exercise 2: Wall reaching exercise. This is done while standing facing a wall with your feet apart and your forehead resting against the wall. Creep your hands up the wall as far as possible, trying to reach higher each day. Mark the place you've reached so that you can aim higher every time. The idea is to be able to stretch your arms up with your elbows straight so that eventually your palms can be brought face to face with each other as in the lower right hand picture.

Exercise 3: Ball on Elastic. Get someone to thread a ball on to a piece of elastic for you. Loop the elastic around the middle finger of the hand on the affected side and throw the ball around in any direction. As you improve you'll be able to catch it at the end of each trajectory but don't worry if you can't do this early on.

Exercise 4: Door and rope exercise. Get a piece of cord or thin rope and tie one end to a door handle and the other to a piece of dowel (a thick pencil will do). Move your arm in small circles from the shoulder while standing a long way from the door. As you improve you can get closer to the door and enlarge your circle size. Don't forget to move your arm both clockwise and anti-clockwise with this exercise.

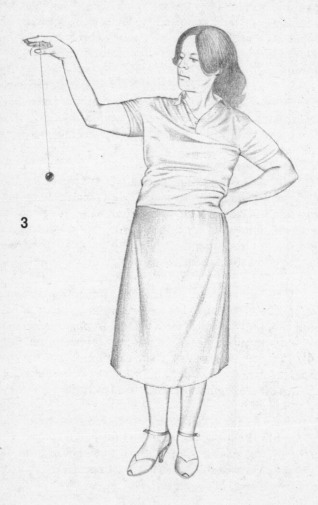

3

Exercise 3.

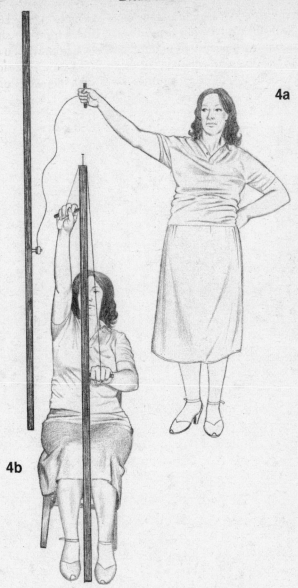

Exercise 4.

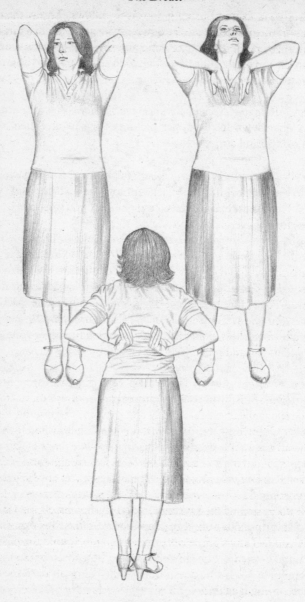

Exercises 5 and 6.

Another good exercise using a door is as follows. Throw the rope over the top of an open door. Sit down as shown in the diagram and then pull the rope first with one hand and then the other as if over a pulley on the top of the door. Use your good arm to pull up the arm on the operated side.

Exercise 5: Relaxing excercise for back and shoulder. Put your arms in the positions shown in the upper pictures opposite and then rotate them clockwise and anti-clockwise.

Exercise 6: Bra fastening. As you begin to improve, repeatedly do up and undo your bra behind your back. Alternatively, do the same with an apron. Once these exercises can easily be done you won't need to do any other formal exercises.

Exercise 7: Deep breathing. Sit down and do the following exercise aimed at improving your posture and the tightness across the chest. Do this exercise frequently, even when you're just sitting down anywhere. Place the hand that feels most comfortable over the centre of your chest. Take a slow deep breath through your nose and really make your chest expand. Exhale completely and let your chest and shoulders sag and relax. Repeat as many times as you can.

Exercise 8: Posture. Always try to keep your shoulders straight and avoid stooping. Most women stoop automatically after a mastectomy, partly to relieve the chest discomfort and partly to disguise the loss of the breast. Unfortunately, drooping the shoulders makes for weak muscles and makes it impossible to maintain a wide range of shoulder movements. Stand in front of your mirror regularly and train yourself to stand well. You'll feel a lot better for this, especially once you have a breast prosthesis.

When doing any of the exercises, never push yourself too far. Do them for short periods at first then gradually try to achieve more and more. If you feel any tightness, pain or discomfort, hold the position in which the discomfort began and do some slow, deep breathing for half a minute or so. If this doesn't dispel the pain wait until the next day before trying it again.

Just because you're going for radiotherapy or other treatments, don't forget to do your exercises, because even though you may feel

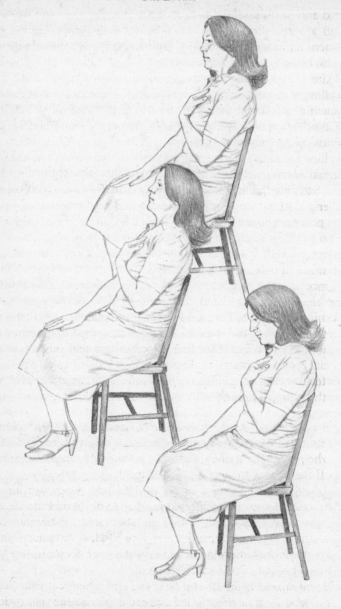

Deep breathing exercise (see page 187 for description).

tired and ill it's essential to keep the whole area loose and free from fluid accumulation. If you don't bother with your excercises permanent limitation of movement can occur, especially if radiotherapy is also being given to the chest area.

After a radical mastectomy about a quarter of women have some swelling of the arm on the operated side. This comes about because by removing the lymph nodes in the armpit the surgeon substantially blocks the flow of lymph and tissue fluid from the arm. This fluid then builds up and makes the arm swell. In only one in ten women is this swelling (oedema) incapacitating. Some swelling occurs in nearly all women immediately post-operatively but this goes within a week or two. Swelling that is still there after two to three weeks will probably never go. Many surgeons have tried to devise the perfect operation that produces no arm swelling at all but it has so far proved impossible to do so. Even aggressive physical treatments from physiotherapists cannot prevent it altogether but sleeping with the arm raised on pillows definitely aids gravity's efforts to drain the fluid from the arm.

Once the swelling is there, relief is not easy to obtain. Some women find that bandaging the arm helps, especially if done early in the morning before it has swollen too much and others use a commercial sleeve pump. Because of the stagnation of the lymph, the affected arm is more liable to infection than the other arm and this means that special care must be taken. About one in ten women who have had a mastectomy will have a finger or hand infected at some time so it's well worth trying to prevent infection occurring. Here are a few useful tips:

1. *Always protect the shoulder, arm and hand on the affected side from burns.* Hold cigarettes in the other hand; wear padded oven gloves when doing the cooking and avoid getting suntanned. Take things off the stove with your uninvolved hand.

2. *Don't constrict the arm on the affected side.* Keep watches and bracelets loose on the affected hand and arm. Avoid dresses with tight sleeves (especially if they are elasticated). Preferably avoid wearing rings on that hand. Carry your handbag or basket with the good arm, not the bad one. Always ask your doctor to take your blood pressure in the unaffected arm.

3. *Avoid injuries to the affected hand and arm.* Don't cut your finger-nails too short on the affected side and don't damage your cuticles. Use a cuticle cream instead of cutting if you need to do anything to

them at all. Use rubber gloves when using steel wool or abrasive pot scourers. Wear rubber or other thick gloves when gardening. Ask doctors to take blood, when necessary, from your other arm. Wear a thimble when sewing and don't prick your finger with needles and pins. Shave under your arms (if you normally do so) with an electric razor to avoid scratches and nicks. Don't have vaccinations done on the affected arm.

4. *Look after minor injuries at once.* If ever you do get a break in the skin, however small, wash it at once with water, use an antiseptic cream and bandage it. Don't use adhesive dressings. Always tell your doctor at once about any swelling, soreness or inflammation. If this occurs, he'll suggest that you elevate the arm. He may also suggest warm soaks and antibiotics. This treatment usually cures the condition in a few days.

A condition called *lymphangitis* can affect the post-mastectomy arm. It shows itself as thin red streaks that extend up the arm and even on to the upper arm. It is an inflammation of the lymphatic channels and is caused by an infection (sometimes unnoticed) in the hand somewhere. Antibiotics and elevation of the arm often cure it quickly.

5. *Don't use the affected arm for heavy work.*

6. *Avoid detergents that cause cracking of the hands or wear rubber gloves.* Infections can get in through cracks. In cold weather use hand lotions or creams regularly.

7. *In general, continue with all your normal activities but with caution based on the above list.* Rest the arm frequently, preferably in a slightly elevated position. Driving can be resumed as soon as your affected arm is strong enough to cope. Lovemaking can be resumed as soon as you feel like it. There is little doubt that getting back to a normal life does wonders for the ego of a woman who has lost her breast, and a loving couple will soon find ways around any temporary discomfort there might be because of the scars and swelling. With these provisos there's no reason why you shouldn't make love the day you get home. In fact there's every reason why you should!

Some women notice a number of very strange phenomena after a mastectomy. One of the commonest is the *phantom breast syndrome*. In this the woman has the sensation that the breast is still there. The most common complaints are of tingling and itching, though burning and a sensation of heaviness are not uncommon. In one study over half of all mastectomy patients had the phantom breast syndrome but the majority hadn't told their doctors. About a fifth of women with this syndrome notice a worsening during the day and a tenth a worsening during the night. It takes more than a week for the symptoms to come on in some women but two-thirds have the sensations within the first week after the operation. One major study found that women who had this syndrome were in general younger and tended to have a lower opinion of their relationship with their husband than older women. They also thought they had poor emotional support from their surgeons and were more likely to have an increased intake of tranquillizers after mastectomy. They also blamed their emotional and social problems on the mastectomy more than did other women.

Reaction to hot and cold drinks is another strange post-mastectomy syndrome that is little spoken of. While drinking very hot or cold drinks a strange sensation is sometimes felt in the area of the scar. As the fluid flows into the stomach the sensations disappear. This is almost certainly caused by the stimulation of a neurological pathway by the hot or cold fluid touching the back of the throat and upper oesophagus. It has no serious significance.

GETTING YOUR SHAPE BACK

If the surgeon has *not* inserted an implant at the time of the operation, and this is most often the case, you'll be given advice on a prosthetic device (a false breast). In the early weeks it's best to use a simple, inexpensive, light-weight, foam rubber pad to fill out your bra on the operated side and this makes most women feel a lot better about having had their breast removed. It's also more comfortable to sleep with a light-weight prosthesis like this in a light sleep bra. About six to eight weeks after the operation, when the area has settled down, you can have a heavier and more realistic breast prosthesis fitted. This can be supplied free on the National Health Service or can be bought from a specialist firm or mastectomy centre. There are seven types of prosthesis available now on the National Health Service so one should suit you. The best ones are made of liquid silicone gel in a silicone bag, are skin-coloured and feel (through a bra) just like a real breast. They come in various sizes, take up the body's temperature and can be washed easily. Most women who have these are extremely pleased with them and people who don't know about their mastectomy are never able to tell that the breast is a false one.

You don't necessarily have to have a special bra after a mastectomy, although your hospital can fit a pocket inside your own bra (free of charge) so that your prosthesis can fit into it. You can buy special swimwear to take a prosthesis but most women find a normal swimsuit is just as good. Any good corsetry fitter will advise you on mastectomy bras and swimwear, or you can get further information from the Mastectomy Association (address below).

THE EMOTIONAL AFTERMATH

Looking normal to outsiders is only a part of coming to terms with a mastectomy and, as with so many medical conditions, people who have been down the same path before can be very helpful. Mastectomy is no exception. The Mastectomy Association, 25 Brighton Road, South Croydon CR2 6EA, Surrey (telephone: 01-654 8643) was started by a mastectomy patient and helps doctors and patients who want to know more about living with a mastectomy. The Association's sensitive and practical advice helps many of the thousands of women who lose a breast every year and this help often extends to their families and medical advisers too. That such an organization is needed can be seen from a recent study which found that one year after surgery for breast cancer a quarter of all women needed treatment for anxiety and depression (compared with 5 per cent of a control group of women with non-cancerous breast lumps). One-third had moderate or severe sexual difficulties (8 per cent in the control group). Sympathetic help from people who have been through the same experience undoubtedly reduces the negative feelings and insecurity experienced by most women at some time after a mastectomy and many find that helping others in a similar situation helps them to come to terms with their own problems.

Once the immediate horrors of the situation are over, worries about sex and sexuality often dominate a woman's emotions after a mastectomy. Many women say that they feel less of a woman and the natural reaction is to feel totally unsexy and undesirable in the early days. Some women even feel strongly enough to say that they'd rather have kept their breast and lived a few years less.

The one key factor that emerges from a lot of research into this subject is that the role of the woman's partner is absolutely crucial.

And this is true of women of all types, levels of intelligence and education. Ideally the woman's husband or lover should be actively involved throughout the whole process right from when the lump is discovered. In this way the woman feels she has the support she needs and does much better.

There is no reason why sexual intercourse shouldn't be resumed the day the woman gets home. There is no such thing as too much sex after a mastectomy and as long as the wound area isn't hurt there are no problems. It's a matter of trial and error to find a position that suits the couple and then to use it until healing is complete.

Some women are afraid that their partners will leave them – the underlying fear being that a woman with one breast won't be able to attract and keep a man. The facts are that the vast majority of men do not leave their woman after a mastectomy and that most worry a lot about how to be supportive and helpful. Although most women try to hide their chests (especially in the early days) from their partners, most men are not as upset by the loss of the breast as women think they'll be.

However, some couples approach a mastectomy with considerable psychosexual and relationship problems already and for them the mastectomy is sometimes the last straw. That this is unusual can be seen from one study which found that two-thirds of post-mastectomy women judged their emotional state to be excellent or very good. Women who fared best had been married longer, had found their partners (and doctors) more supportive and were pleased with the response from their children and the hospital staff.

Strange as it may seem, most women say that the worst time emotionally is immediately after the lump is discovered. Only one in seven women in one study found the immediate post-operative period the most difficult. Although most women have thoughts about mutilation, loss of femininity and death, several studies have found that the good news outweighs the bad. One study, for example, found that 71 per cent of women rated their husband's reactions to the mastectomy as extremely or very understanding; 76 per cent felt that the loss of the breast made no difference or had a positive effect on their sexual satisfaction or their ability to be orgasmic; and 60 per cent rated their overall post-mastectomy adjustment as very good.

Many women have married after a mastectomy. If you are still having periods, you may find you'll get the same sort of discomfort on your mastectomy side that you would normally get in both breasts at this time of the month.

Remember that talking about it with your husband, family and friends is bound to help. Slowly they'll all come to terms with your new condition.

Up to here we have talked about the woman who will return to normal health after her operation. Unfortunately a small proportion of women will have such advanced disease, even before first seeing their doctor, that by the time surgery is done they are in a very bad physical state and will need other non-surgical treatments (see below). The goal for such women is for them to maintain their independence, physical activity and work levels in the best possible way they can. Research in a London teaching hospital has found that women who keep optimistic, cheerful and positive, even in the face of their killing disease, do better and actually live longer than women who give up and resign themselves to death. In fact many people who work with cancer patients of all kinds say how remarkable it is that some seem to 'will' themselves to live while others 'put their face to the wall' and wait for death. There is absolutely no doubt that one's psychological attitude can considerably alter one's outlook with breast cancer and current research is finding that the body's immune system can be altered for the worse in people under stress. It is increasingly being maintained that the body's natural anti-cancer surveillance system is boosted in those people who have a positive will to live.

Once the disease has reached a terminal stage, medical and social care are aimed at keeping the woman pain-free and at home with her family for as long as possible.

Treatments other than surgery for breast cancer

Basically there are few other types of treatment that can be used in breast cancer. They can be used before and/or after surgery but are usually used afterwards. There is, as we saw on page 173, little agreement among experts as to what is the ideal treatment for breast cancer and the combinations of surgery and any of the four treatments outlined below that you receive will depend on your surgeon and the nature of your condition. Confusingly, treatment methods even vary from surgeon to surgeon within any one unit.

RADIOTHERAPY

Radiotherapy (the therapeutic use of irradiation) is a very vexed subject when it comes to treating breast cancer. It was often used post-operatively as a routine measure to try to kill off any remaining cancer cells in the breast and surrounding areas once the lump had been removed. Research has shown that such routine radiotherapy doesn't improve survival figures so it's now used only in selected cases known to respond. This is just as well because although it's completely painless at the time a skin burn (like sunburn) develops over the treated area and can be unpleasant. The X-rays used also kill normal cells and the patient may become more sensitive to infections and may suffer inflammation of bones and joints. Apart from the pain, the local changes in the chest skin often mean that a woman can't wear a prosthesis as early as she otherwise could and this is often distressing in itself. Some women also have some shortness of breath or a cough as a result of the X-ray effects on the underlying lung but this is neither a serious nor a permanent side-effect. The dose has to be carefully calculated as radiotherapy can prevent wounds healing, especially after a mastectomy when flaps of skin with a poor blood supply are pulled tightly together.

It's difficult to predict how any given woman's tissues will react to radiation. Sometimes the treatment produces no side-effects while in others there is considerable fibrosis which shows itself as a thickening of the area being treated. Many women develop fine blood vessel dilatations called spider naevi. These are completely harmless and disappear quickly. In the past, the results of radiotherapy were not so good and the dose used often caused unsightly scarring in the remaining breast tissue. Today though this is very uncommon indeed.

A variation of radiotherapy has come from France. In it, radiotherapy is combined with radiation from iridium wires inserted into the breast. This treatment appears to be at least as effective as radical mastectomy in controlling the cancer and produces a better effect aesthetically. In half of all cases the breast has a completely normal appearance after treatment; in others there are alterations but the patients are still pleased with the results. A similar method is now being tried by several USA centres, including Yale and Harvard.

CHEMOTHERAPY

Chemotherapy is the name given to treatment with anti-cancer (cytotoxic) drugs. The concept of a drug to *cure* cancer is an attractive one but the reality is, alas, a long way off. Cancer cells, unlike bacteria which are foreign to the body, are simply normal cells that have gone wrong. This means that in order to kill them one has to tread a fine line to avoid killing off normal cells too. Drugs used to be tried only in the most hopeless cases of breast cancer but even then there were no true 'cures'. Today they are sometimes used earlier on in a preventive way but most doctors still keep them as a last resort.

The use of anti-cancer drugs is very controversial and their side effects can be unpleasant. Tolerance to them varies enormously from woman to woman and it is often difficult for the surgeon to obtain the desired results without producing any side effects. Several of the anti-cancer drugs immobilize the woman's infection-fighting ability and she is therefore susceptible to the most minor of infections. Some of the drugs make the hair fall out but many women are happy to put up with this and wear a wig if the drug is curing the cancer. Other side effects include violent nausea and diarrhoea and there could be more serious long-term effects. The British Breast Group (a body of doctors with a special interest in breast cancer) recommends that drugs like this should only be used when the cancer has definitely spread beyond the breast. Side effects are generally only a nuisance (as opposed to life-threatening) but even so, many women are not prepared to put up with them.

At present there is no single drug or even group of drugs that can be said to be specifically active in breast cancer but good results can be obtained in those cancers that recur after other forms of treatment. Chemotherapy rarely actually *cures* the cancer: it is usually only palliative. Some centres use *adjuvant chemotherapy* which entails giving the drugs fairly soon after the initial treatment for the cancer. This is meant to be prophylactic (preventive) and is aimed at preventing recurrences before they get a foothold. Results with such a regime are confused and it is by no means a proven way of preventing recurrences.

HORMONE THERAPY

We have seen in several parts of the book that some breast cancers seem to be hormone-dependent and we saw on page 176 that surgical removal of certain of the hormone-producing glands in the body can produce promising results in the disease. In very recent years though the whole subject has taken an interesting turn with the discovery of hormone receptors in breast tissue.

Normal tissues, including those of the breast, often have specific substances within their cells or on their cell walls that attract and hold on to specific hormones. These binding areas are called receptor sites and only if they are there can particular hormones have an effect on that cell. Breast tissue contains oestrogen receptors, for example, and when malignant cells develop in the breast they may or may not still have the receptor system. If a cancer keeps the receptor mechanism it tends to be oestrogen-dependent and behaves rather differently from one that has no oestrogen receptors. It has been postulated that breast tumours are of three basic kinds: those that rely on hormones for survival; those that react to hormones; and those that aren't affected at all by hormones.

It is now possible to tell the difference between such tumours and to use the information clinically. Several procedures are available to measure oestrogen receptors in normal and diseased breast tissue. A sample of tissue is taken, frozen quickly and then tested. If the tests show that the tumour is oestrogen-responsive it can be treated with anti-oestrogens (tamoxifen, clomiphene and amino-glutethimide) and such trials are currently under way. In certain centres such drugs are being used alongside chemotherapy.

Our understanding of all this is in its very early stages but it does seem clear that women with high levels of oestrogen receptors will respond to some kind of hormonal therapy if their cancers recur and that such treatment is worth considering before chemotherapy is started. If the tumour has no oestrogen receptors, on the other hand, it makes sense to go straight to other treatments if the tumour recurs and not to waste time on hormonal ones.

IMMUNOTHERAPY

It is now widely accepted that our bodies have a surveillance system that usually recognizes tumour cells as they arise and deals with them through the immune (antigen-antibody) system of the body. Sometimes this system doesn't function and the person is predisposed to getting cancer. There are no definite advances in this area worth reporting but a lot of research is going on into three main areas. First, it may be possible to immunize a woman against her own cancer cells but this hasn't proved to be valuable so far in breast cancer; second, it might be possible to boost the body's immune defence system somehow; and third, it might be possible to produce a kind of passive immunization (using cells or serum from a woman already immunized against breast cancer). This latter technique has not yet proved valuable with breast cancer.

The drug levamisole and the anti-tuberculous vaccine BCG boost the body's immune response and giving these drugs has resulted in the reduction of tumour growth in some people. Unfortunately, women with breast cancer don't seem to respond well to these drugs.

Recurrences

Some women will develop a local or distant recurrence of their cancer within a few years of the original surgery. Most such recurrences occur within the first seven years but some women only have trouble twenty years later. No one knows why this should be but it is thought that the cancer cells lie dormant and then regrow.

Any woman who has had a breast cancer is about twice as likely to suffer another growth in the opposite breast. This means that such women should take great care to feel their other breast every month and go for regular checkups by their doctor. Some surgeons suggest a twice-yearly follow up almost indefinitely for such women (assuming they are completely cured of their first tumour). Some surgeons even go so far as to do random biopsies of the other breast but this is not common.

Apart from recurrences (or new primary growths) in the other breast, they can also occur under the skin of the operated side. Such local recurrences can be excised at an operation or treated with X-ray therapy.

The outcome

The first question many women have once the diagnosis has been made is, 'How long have I got to live?' Unfortunately even with all our sophisticated tests and knowledge today there is no way of answering the question. Although there are certain guidelines (see below), nature fools us every day of the week and it is a foolish surgeon who tells a woman how long she'll survive. After all, the statistics are the result of studying and analysing many thousands of women in any given situation. Within any one such group, the spread of results can be enormous. It is therefore almost impossible to give a prognosis (outlook) for any given woman although it is probably fair to try to do so for her tumour. Thankfully the two are not the same and, as we have seen, a woman can substantially modify her outlook by her attitude to the disease.

Here are some guidelines as to the outcome for women with breast cancers.

1. There is little doubt that lumps discovered when they are small have a better outlook than those discovered when large.
2. The longer the interval between the time of discovery and the start of treatment, the worse the outlook.
3. Cancers in the outer third of the breast seem to do better than those placed centrally.
4. Tumours centred on the duct system of the breast seem to do better than those that have spread throughout the breast.
5. Cancers in one place in the breast do better than those that are spread over many sites within the breast.
6. Tumours that are confined solely to the breasts have a better outlook than those that have spread elsewhere (even to the lymph nodes).
7. The presence of certain cellular components called Barr bodies (seen around the outer rim of cancer cells) indicates a good prognosis, especially if more than half of the cells have these structures.
8. If the level of oestrogen receptors in the breast cancer tissue is low, the outlook is good.

Breast cancer is an emotive and unpleasant disease. It is no more common than it has been for several decades but the outlook for the woman who contracts the disease is not much better than it would have been ten or fifteen years ago. However, although most women will live no longer with their disease than they would have done a decade ago, today's treatments are less unpleasant and the quality of their remaining life is rather higher than it used to be.

If the amount of money and research that is being poured into breast cancer research is anything to go by there should be some more hopeful news to report within a very few years.

CHAPTER 9

Cosmetic surgery
and other ways of changing your breasts

As we found in our survey, a substantial proportion of women say they are dissatisfied with their breasts. Indeed it is uncommon to meet a woman who *is* totally satisfied with her breasts. We have seen in other parts of the book why this dissatisfaction has come about but in this chapter we're going to see what can be done to help a woman to improve on what nature gave her.

Because many women are so insecure about their breasts they are wide open to exploitation by unscrupulous people who promise great things. Bust developers, creams, exercisers and water splash equipment are bought by countless thousands of women every year the world over yet there is absolutely no evidence that they do anything to enlarge the breast (which is what they are usually bought for). Hormone creams, tablets, injections, massages and so on are also available commercially but are all equally ineffective. Hormone creams containing oestrogens work for as long as you keep using them but the hormones are absorbed through the skin and have generalized effects in the body. There has been enough publicity about the negative effects of high-oestrogen contraceptive pills to put most thinking women off using such creams. Some of these methods can produce a moderate bust enlargement over a long period by suggestion, as we shall see later in this chapter, but even this is uncommon. Twenty-six per cent of the women in our survey had tried methods of bust enlargement and 5 per cent thought that what they had tried worked. The fact that some methods, shown in trials to be useless, work for some women perhaps simply proves the power of suggestion (see page 206).

Most women who are dissatisfied with their breasts believe they are too small and therefore unattractive. As a result, most of the gadgets, creams, operations and so on are geared to bust enlargement. Padded bras are the most popular way of making a bust look bigger than it really is but in this chapter we're going to look at things that might actually increase breast size and not at ways of fooling onlookers. There are only two things that have been proven to enlarge the breasts. One other simply enlarges the muscles underneath and makes the breasts *seem* bigger. Let's look at each in turn.

Enlarging your breasts

EXERCISES

As we saw in Chapter 3 the breasts sit on two muscles that in turn lie on the chest wall. These muscles are attached at one end to the chest and at the other to the arm and shoulder. Enlarging these muscles by exercising them makes them more bulky and pushes forward what breast tissue there is, so making the breasts appear bigger. Any exercises that increase the bulk of these pectoral muscles will make the breasts seem bigger if they are done often enough and for long enough.

Here are two useful exercises. Stand with your arms bent at breast level, thumbs against your chest, and make quick, short pulling movements backwards as if attempting to make your elbows meet

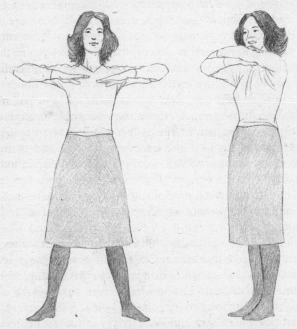

Two exercises for enlarging the muscles that lie under the breasts.

between your shoulderblades. Repeat this twenty to thirty times at least once a day.

In the second exercise you fold your arms in front of you with your hands gripping your arms just above the elbows. Now push your hands against your arms and you'll feel the muscles under your breasts jump. Do this at least twenty to thirty times, preferably morning and night.

COSMETIC SURGERY

In our Western society many women see themselves as being inadequate and possibly even sexually unacceptable if their breasts are small. For some the feelings are so great that they are prepared to undergo in-patient surgical procedures to remedy their 'problems'.

Before the current vogue for and expertise in plastic surgery other methods of surgical breast enlargement were tried all over the world. Liquid paraffin first came into use about the time of World War I. At this time paraffin was being used for both facial wrinkles and enlarging the breast. At first the injection of this fluid, and seemingly inert, substance appeared to produce no problems but quite soon it became apparent that many women developed non-malignant tumours (paraffinomas) where the paraffin was injected.

Silicones were next tried because they could be produced as low viscosity fluids or high viscosity semi-solid gels. Fluid silicone found its way into the hands of many unqualified practitioners, some of whom mixed it with oils (olive oil was commonly used) so as to produce local inflammation which in turn would induce fibrous tissue formation and so seal off the silicone within the breast. Silicone injections were fraught with problems, though. The liquid started to 'travel' within the breast, could be accidentally injected into blood vessels and could produce breast cysts. The results overall were disastrous and many women the world over have ended up having their breasts removed because of the deformities and ulceration caused by silicone. Injectable silicone is now banned in the USA and is scarcely used anywhere in the Western world.

Fat-dermal grafts were another surgical approach that was tried. In this procedure a chunk of fat and skin was removed from the buttock (leaving the scar in the fold under the buttock) and was inserted under the breast through an incision under it. The initial results were often very good but over the months the fat tended to liquefy and be absorbed. The scarred fat and dermis left a nodular appearance and the woman was usually disappointed.

After World War II plastics began to come on the scene and many surgeons experimented with breast implants cut out of lumps of various plastics. Unfortunately these, and sponge prostheses, all had the disadvantage of causing fibrous tissue to form around them and they soon became walled off and very hard to the touch.

Today's plastic surgery has come a long way from all of these procedures. The considerable interest shown by women in the Western world (and especially in the USA) has meant that time, research and money have been invested in the subject and today's results are excellent and usually without complications in good hands. The suffering today is usually only financial!

The most commonly used surgical method of enlarging the breast today is the insertion of a silicone bag filled with silicone gel behind the breast through an incision made under the breast. Early types of implant had a Dacron backing which helped fix the prosthesis to the chest wall but today's implants are simply put in place and left there. Many surgeons have experimented with inflatable implants over the years because being smaller (in the deflated form) they could be inserted through a very small incision. They are blown up to the desired size when in place. These inflatable models haven't caught on, though, mainly because they can deflate and can be ruptured.

Some surgeons advise women over the age of thirty-five to have a mammogram (see page 150) before their operation, just in case there is a lump. After all, breast cancer is relatively common and it would be terrible to undergo cosmetic surgery on the breast only to have to have it removed some months or even years later.

The operation to insert a silicone implant is simple and can be done under a local or (more usually) a general anaesthetic. Some surgeons make the incision in the fold under the breast and others insert the prosthesis through an incision around the areola. Whichever approach is used the breast is lifted away from the underlying muscle to create a space large enough to receive a suitably sized implant. Some surgeons are experimenting with the insertion of the implant through an incision under the armpit. Whenever possible both breasts are operated upon at the same time. The operation takes about one and a half hours per breast, depending on what is to be done.

A woman who has such an operation is up and about the same day (some centres in the USA do the whole thing as an out-patient procedure), and usually has little or no discomfort. Bleeding into the breast is the only immediate possible complication and this can be dangerous because a pool of blood there can become infected. This greatly increases the likelihood that the implant will be rejected. About 10 to 15 per cent of women have some kind of complaint (be it medical or aesthetic) after these procedures. A breast augmentation operation carried out under general anaesthetic carries the same risks from the anaesthetic and other factors as does any operation.

The only long-term complication that occurs is the development of a firm or hard breast. Between 20 and 40 per cent of all women having an implant will complain of one or other breast becoming hard some months after the operation. This arises because the silicone, recognized by the body as 'foreign', produces a walling-off reaction in the breast. The tough fibrous tissue that forms makes the breast unacceptably firm to many women and their partners. There is no way of avoiding this problem (which often only affects one side, for some unknown reason). Steroids injected locally at the time of the operation, wearing a bra continuously, the use of exercises after wound healing, and the use of tight dressings have all been tried but with no success. Recently some surgeons have been placing the implant behind the chest muscle to avoid capsule formation.

The capsule of fibrous tissue can be removed surgically at another operation but often recurs. Other ways of overcoming the problem involve rupturing the fibrous capsule. This can be done either by the surgeon or by the woman's partner. Early signs of hardening can be coped with by the woman squeezing the affected breast very hard from time to time. Alternatively, either under an anaesthetic or simply in the clinic a surgeon can perform a sort of nutcracker squeeze with his hands to break down the hard capsule. Unfortunately, it is possible to rupture the implant itself if this is done too vigorously.

Most women who have had this operation are pleased with it. In fact it is the most pleasing cosmetic operation on the breasts. It's important to remember though that you can't be made any size you choose – the surgeon can only insert the size of implant that will fit behind your breast. In general it's wisest to settle for something smaller than you first think you'd like. The results are then better and you'll look more natural. Also if your breasts started off being unequal the insertion of an implant could well emphasize the difference. Some-

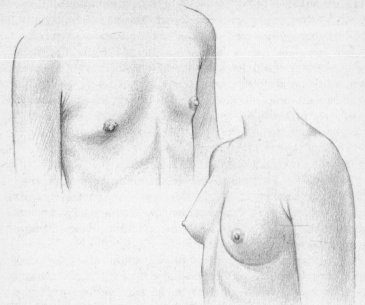

A woman before and after a breast enlargement operation.

times a surgeon will place different-sized implants under each breast so as to match up the sizes.

In the immediate post-operative period (say two to three weeks) it makes sense to wear a snugly fitting bra and some surgeons suggest that the woman should manipulate her breasts several times a day to discourage the formation of the fibrous capsule. To do this the woman pushes both breasts firmly towards one another and then upwards, outwards and finally downwards. This can be repeated about ten times several times a day. It probably makes sense not to raise the arms fully above the head or to lift things in the few weeks immediately following the implant because this can slow the process which fixes the prosthesis to the chest wall and it can then slip.

A later problem can occur if a woman who has had an implant becomes pregnant. The heavier, swollen breast of pregnancy may sag into a very unfortunate shape unless supported with a well-fitting bra.

Whilst silicone gel implants are successful in enlarging an otherwise small breast, they are not good for misshapen or sagging breasts. These deformities can be corrected in other ways, as we shall see.

There is no evidence that the use of these implants increase the risks of getting breast cancer and most women who have had the operation will be able to breastfeed. For the first two weeks after surgery the nipple and areola have reduced sensation and can take many months to return to normal. One study found that one in seven women still had sensation losses two years after the procedure, especially those who had large implants inserted. The skin over the rest of the breast returned to normal far more quickly and nipple erectability and sensuality returned much earlier than did sensation.

HYPNOSIS AND VISUAL IMAGERY

It has been known for thousands of years that it is possible to alter basic body functions using only the mind. Yogis can train themselves to control certain functions of their internal organs and research shows that most of us can be trained to change the blood flow to specific areas of the body at will.

This knowledge, and a desire to save women the minor, though rare, dangers inherent in any operation, led several USA researchers to look at the possibilities of enlarging the breasts using visual imagery and other similar techniques. In one study twenty-two volunteers ranging in age from nineteen to fifty-four were taught to hypnotize themselves and to use visual imagery to increase their breast size. Using cassette tapes, the subjects were asked to visualize a wet, warm towel over their breasts and to allow this to produce a feeling of warmth. As soon as they could feel the warmth over their breasts they were asked to concentrate on a feeling of pulsation in the breasts, to become aware of their heartbeat and to 'allow the heartbeat to flow' into their breasts. They were then instructed to practise this imagery while relaxing at home once a day. On the initial visit each subject was hypnotized and helped to relax.

At the end of twelve weeks nearly one third of the women had reached their ideal bust size they had set before the programme started and said that they wanted no further enlargement. Nearly half of all the women had to buy a bigger bra. Forty-two per cent lost weight during the programme yet still had breast enlargement. But most encouraging of all was that three-quarters of the women noted positive changes in their lives while taking part in the study. At the end of twelve weeks 85 per cent of the volunteers could obtain a spontaneous feeling of warmth and pulsation in their breasts just by thinking about it even while driving, watching television or at work. Those women who could easily and quickly obtain visual imagery did best and arrived at their desired breast size quickest.

Just why this method (since repeated in other studies) works, is not clear. It has been suggested that the mechanism might be hormonal because it is known that the emotions can influence hormone production. There is some evidence that disruptive and negative emotional environments can adversely affect the development of breasts during adolescence. In one case, a girl of fifteen years was found to be small in stature and to have no secondary sexual characteristics (pubic and axillary hair, breasts etc) at all. She was removed from her poor environment and after six weeks had developed breasts and put on one inch in height. Over the next eight months she had grown four inches, had substantial breast development and pubic hair.

Another theory as to why the hypnosis method might work is that the breasts simply become engorged with blood. This could explain the finding in another study that breast size at a three-month follow up had diminished from the immediate post-treatment level, but even so more than three-quarters of the gain in size remained.

Clearly such a technique needs ideally to be taught by someone experienced in hypnotherapy but there is no doubt that many women who are good at visual imagery could use this technique themselves at home. It's almost certainly completely harmless and is a lot easier and cheaper than an operation.

Reducing breast-size

It is ironic that women with tiny breasts envy those with large ones and vice versa but perhaps this is simply a manifestation of 'the other woman's grass is always greener' syndrome. Women with small breasts may have psychological or sexual problems but women with very large breasts often also have very real physical problems to add to these.

The story of the woman with very large breasts is usually that they enlarged rapidly during adolesence and that since then they have made her life a misery. She cannot buy large enough bras or dresses; her bra straps cut into her shoulders causing chafing, pigmentation or actual bleeding; she gets sore underneath the breasts where sweat accumulates; she gets pain in her back and shoulders; she walks with a rounded back; and she may even have pains, numbness or tingling in her hands and forearms.

Jogging and playing games are avoided because of the discomfort and many daily tasks are difficult, if not impossible, because the breast mass makes arm and shoulder movement difficult. Some women go on a weight-reducing diet only to find that they lose weight from the rest of their body leaving their breasts looking relatively even larger. There is usually no breast pain with this condition — indeed the opposite is often the case, with women complaining of a lack of sensation and certainly very little, if any, erotic pleasure from their breasts.

In the past it was usually women over forty who sought help with this problem but today girls in their teens are asking for help. Most surgeons won't consider reducing the breasts until full body growth has stopped, in the early twenties.

While very large breasts have no greater susceptibility to cancer, there is no doubt that both doctors and women themselves find it much more difficult to feel such breasts for lumps. This means that a lump could grow to a much larger size than would be possible in a small-breasted woman before it was noticed. This is another reason why many women want to have their large breasts reduced in size.

No one knows why some women's breasts become so large. There seems to be a familial tendency but this is not a consistent finding. Hormones have been blamed but no hormone therapy can cure large breasts.

Many women ask their plastic surgeon to 'make me as small as you can' or words to that effect, simply because they are overreacting to the horrors of their deformity. Surgeons, knowing this, will usually go for a B or C (rather than an A) cup, having learned from experience that this is what is most satisfactory for the woman in the long run.

Operations to reduce the breast are more complex than those to augment it. Quite simply all the methods aim at reducing the amount of breast tissue (which in these women is composed mainly of fat) and to make a new 'skin brassière'. There are two main techniques. In one, the nipple, attached to a piece of breast tissue, is transferred to a new site and in the other it is removed completely and re-sited. Both procedures reduce nipple sensation and when the nipple is removed and re-sited there is often no sensation at all for up to two years. In the more usual operation in which the areola and nipple are lifted and kept on a stalk of tissue there is less loss of sensation but many women say they are still insensitive after six months. One study found that breast sensation had returned in 65 per cent of women tested two years after the operation. Sensation on the skin over the rest of the breast returns before that of the nipple and areola and in both types of operation the nipple responds to sexual arousal much earlier than to touch or pain sensations. The larger the breast, the more tissue has to be removed and the more is the sensation loss in general.

Before the operation the surgeon will draw the outline of the ideal 'finished' position of the breast with a felt tip pen. The operation is then done under general anaesthesia and the woman's appearance checked sitting up while she is still under the anaesthetic. A large dressing is applied to reduce the amount of internal bleeding and a suction or other drain may be left in the breast for a few days to help any leaking tissue fluid and blood to drain freely. This reduces the likelihood of post-operative infection. Most women are home again within a week after the surgery.

With most of the operations there is a T-shaped incision running from the nipple to the fold under the breast. The base of the T-shape is at the nipple and the cross piece in the fold.

The scars are, unfortunately, often troublesome and some widening of the vertical part of the T often occurs. On occasions it will be

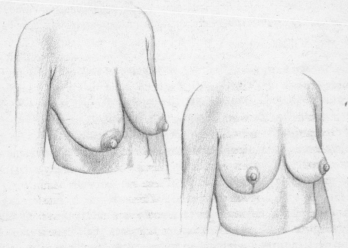

A woman before and after breast reduction surgery.

necessary to re-operate (possibly under local anaesthesia) to improve on the scars.

Most women are pleased with their breast reduction, especially if they have been dogged by physical symptoms for some years. Relatively little tissue is in fact removed – usually about ½-1 kg (1-2 lb) per breast – though rarely, as much as 4½-5½ kg (10-12 lb) has to be removed from each breast. Breastfeeding may be possible afterwards as the ducts may recanalize.

Apart from occasional problems with wound healing there are several other long-term troubles after breast reduction, the commonest of which is fat necrosis. In some women the fat in the operated breast breaks down and this can lead to infection. If a lot of liquefaction occurs the breasts can become unequal and may need another operation later. If the nipple and areola are very large the areola can be trimmed at the same operation to make it more in proportion to the new breast. Some women don't end up with a very pleasing result. Nipple retraction, abnormal pointing of the nipple and asymmetry of the breasts are relatively common and a good surgeon will explain what can go wrong before you agree to the operation.

dressing in place and to support the whole breast but once healing is complete there is no reason why you shouldn't go bra-less from time to time.

Breasts of different sizes

Many women (44 per cent in our survey) have breasts of unequal size but in the vast majority the difference is so small that it doesn't matter to them. Some, however, have discrepancies which show through their clothes even after padding the smaller side. For these women an implant on the smaller side or a reduction of the larger side can provide the answer to their problem.

Pendulous breasts

As a woman ages, her breasts tend to become more pendulous, hanging as much as 15-20 cm (6-8 inches) below their normal position – even though they are not especially big. Because so many women find this unattractive they seek help from plastic surgeons.

They feel and look fine in a bra but don't like what they see when they're not. Exercises are unhelpful. The operations to correct this condition don't remove any breast tissue, only skin. The surgeon forms a new 'skin brassiére' and repositions the nipple aesthetically. Sometimes, once they've been suspended, the breasts look too small and some women decide to have an implant to fill them out. The insertion of implants alone is no good at all for pendulous breasts. Many of those having surgery for pendulous breasts also have a lot of stretch marks, especially on the upper part of the breasts. Unfortunately, although a lot of redundant skin is removed the stretch marks usually remain. There really is no satisfactory treatment for stretch marks on the breasts.

Scars and burns

Some women have had a breast biopsy, have burned their breasts, or have suffered from other kinds of damage to the breast skin. Whenever possible a surgeon makes his incision to remove a lump (or for any other purpose) in a curved parallel to the margin of the areola. Scars that run at right angles to this line can be very unsightly. Often a lump or cyst right out at the edge of the breast is difficult to reach with an ideal incision, and a cross-ways one has to be used.

When wounds heal on the breast they seem to be more likely to produce thickened, pigmented scars called keloids than if elsewhere on the body. Keloids can be removed but in about half of those operated upon the problem recurs.

Breast reconstruction after mastectomy

There is no doubt that the surgeon's first duty when performing a mastectomy must be to remove the tumour as thoroughly as possible, but it is increasingly commonplace to do less and less mutilating operations and to give some thought to the woman's quality of life once her breast has been removed. This has led (as we saw on page 175) to the operation known as subcutaneous mastectomy — a procedure that enables a surgeon to insert a silicone implant either at the original mastectomy operation or later. In the USA especially, many women are consulting a plastic surgeon before their mastectomy to see if something can be done by careful pre-planning. If a woman goes into the operating theatre for a mastectomy knowing that she can and will have a new breast constructed, her whole outlook will be very different. It has been estimated that more than three-quarters of all women having mastectomies come to terms with their post-operative state quite well but that one in five finds it almost impossible to live without a breast. Only a tiny fraction of these eventually have reconstructive surgery.

Even the best possible reconstructions after a mastectomy aren't anywhere like as good as the original breast and often the best that can be achieved is a mound. Still, this is more than acceptable to some women and together with a new nipple (grafted using skin from the other nipple or from the skin of the vulva) the effect can be a very good 'second best'. A woman who has had such an operation may not need to wear a prosthesis and may get away with a padded bra on that side.

Older methods involved the transplanting of tissue from elsewhere in the body but today a silicone implant is almost always used because it doesn't involve the loss of tissue from another part of the body, which itself can be unsightly. Some surgeons use the two and swing a piece of back muscle to cover an implant.

The more radical mastectomies of the past left little skin with which to cover an implant but today's procedures are less destructive and a fair-sized implant can often be covered adequately if it is planned for at the time of the mastectomy. Although the implant can be placed at the time of the mastectomy it is more usual to wait about six months until the skin moves freely over the chest wall. At the operation the surgeon inserts the biggest prosthesis he can (without putting too much strain on the overlying skin) and can even re-operate to insert a larger one months or years later once the skin has stretched a little.

Except in women with very small breasts the new mound will never look like the remaining breast so some surgeons suggest reducing the remaining breast to equalize the woman's appearance. In this way far better symmetry is obtainable. Some surgeons, aware that the other breast of a woman who has had a cancer is at greater risk than the breasts of women who haven't had breast cancer, remove both breasts and do a reconstruction on both sides.

A reconstructed breast doesn't 'flow' normally but stays fixed no matter what you are doing. This is another reason for doing something to equalize both breasts if the woman isn't to look and feel strange.

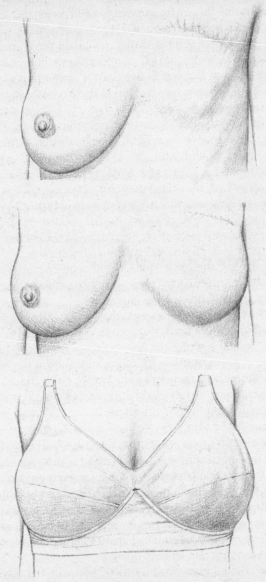

An example of breast reconstruction. *Top:* the appearance after mastectomy; *Middle:* after reconstruction; *Bottom:* the final result in a bra.

Having said all this though, we repeat that a surgeon's first priority *must* be to remove all the tumour and any other tissues he thinks might be affected by it. This means unfortunately that many women simply do not have enough skin left to be able to cover an implant. But 'better be flat-chested and alive rather than a good-looking corpse' must remain the guiding principle for both surgeons and their patients.

Cosmetic surgery of any kind should only be carried out by doctors with a lot of experience, preferably working in a good medical centre or hospital. There are far too many disaster stories around from women who have paid a lot of money only to end up with very unsatisfactory results. Scrupulous control of infection and bleeding are essential for good results and these can best be achieved in highly professional surroundings and by experienced operators. In Britain, if you want to be sure of getting the best possible plastic surgery, discuss the matter with your general practitioner.

Breast surgery for psychological reasons

Not all women with very large or very small breasts have problems that are severe enough to make them want surgery but those that do often have other underlying problems that push them over the brink of accepting what they have. It would be unfair to suggest that all or even most women undergoing plastic surgery on their breasts have psychological or emotional problems but many certainly do. Plastic surgeons have become so used to the woman who thinks a new-look bust will help save her marriage or will lift her flagging self-image after her husband's affair that they take great pains to ensure that a woman's motives are right. Some young women blame their breasts for their lack of success with men but they would get more benefit and suffer fewer hazards if they were to go for psychotherapy rather than plastic surgery! There is a very real danger that if the surgical result is not as good as was hoped for, the neurotic or unstable woman might be severely affected and might have her one remaining excuse for her feelings removed. After such an unsuccessful operation the woman could then be shown up for what she is – a neurotic or disturbed personality – but now with an attractive bust.

However, the small-breasted woman *can* be made to feel inadequate and neurotic by her condition, as one Danish study found. The researchers discovered that there was a fairly consistent psychological picture in the very small-breasted woman. Many were very shy, had given up sports at an early age (mainly to avoid being seen naked in public), had difficulties buying clothes, disliked buying bras, tried to hide their breasts in sexual situations and had suffered scorn and teasing from their contemporaries. This study found that external circumstances usually pushed such women to seek breast enlargement. Divorce, sexual disappointments and new acquaintances were the commonest triggers.

When the women in this study were rated on standard personality scales, 70 per cent were found to have neurotic or hysterical personalities. Their relationships with people were inhibited, remote and rather childish and they were very dependent and felt unsure of themselves. At one year after breast enlargement all the patients were more self-confident and happier with other people. Some said how pleased they were that their bra problems were over and others said how they had gone to 'topless' beaches and enjoyed it. Most were more contact-seeking and interacted better with others.

Other studies of women who had undergone breast enlargement have found that their sex lives often improved. Some women even claim to have expereinced orgasms for the first time as a result of the operation.

Interestingly, husbands in one study were found to be opposed to surgery when the subject was first brought up and some actually said that they feared their wives would be more attractive to other men. In this piece of research the motivating force behind seeking surgery was always the woman, who was self-conscious about her breasts, had little sexual pleasure from them, never undressed in front of men and always made love in the dark. These workers claimed that sexual problems were common in their small-breasted women. All these women were pleased with their operation and told how they frequently examined and admired themselves in the first month after the operation. Breast play, initially limited because of tenderness, increased greatly after the first month and many of the women said that they enjoyed breast sensations for the first time in their lives. They almost all said that they enjoyed being seen naked and that their interest in sex and their intercourse rates rose. Even after three months when the novelty had worn off they all experienced increased self-esteem and happiness. Breast play was still increasing in frequency but intercourse rates were back to the pre-operative level.

Clothing, which for a time had been chosen immediately post-operatively to accentuate the breasts, was back to normal for that particular woman. Most women had incorporated the implant into their body image within sixty days but this took longer if there were post-operative complications.

That breast augmentation has positive psychological and emotional effects on those women who have it cannot be denied. Every parameter of sex (frequency, quality, interest etc) improves dramatically after the procedure. There is no doubt that in a breast-orientated society some women with small breasts are unable to express their true sexuality. It is, however, equally true that millions of women around the world have tiny breasts yet enjoy them and have perfectly happy sexual relationships. The difference between the two groups probably lies in their self image which in turn dates back to their upbringing, especially around the time their breasts were developing.

The overall results of plastic surgery on the breasts are very good indeed and there are lots of satisfied 'customers' around. The results are usually permanent, though the normal breast changes that occur with ageing still take place of course. Only large gains in weight seem to have deleterious effects on otherwise successful surgical procedures.

Most women are out of hospital within a week at the most and can resume sex as soon as they like. Breast play should be gentle or completely curtailed until the wounds are perfectly healed but after this there is no danger to the breast from even quite rough handling. Normal bathing can be resumed within ten to fourteen days and housework after a month. Older women do just as well as younger ones after cosmetic breast operations.

Just because a woman has had a cosmetic operation on her breasts doesn't mean she can ignore her usual monthly self-examination or regular medical checkups. Such breast surgery does nothing one way or the other to one's chances of getting a breast lump and one has to be as vigilant as ever.

Beauty and the breast

Beauty, they say, is in the eyes of the beholder and never was this more true than for a woman's breasts. Much has been written about bust care and a great deal of nonsense has been instilled into women by popular books and magazines, often written by people who are repeating half-baked myths they've heard somewhere.

There is no doubt that a woman who has a good body image and enjoys her femaleness will enjoy her breasts as a part of the whole picture. Good posture, avoiding rounded shoulders, helps make the most of any bust and also makes the whole woman appear more confident. It also shows off her clothes better and this can do wonders for any woman. So quite simply, a woman who likes her body will be happy with her breasts and won't want to or need to do anything to 'improve' them.

However, many women are insecure about their breasts and want to improve things using simple, harmless daily routines that make them feel better. Here are some basic rules to follow so as to keep your breasts looking and feeling good.

1. Always wear a well-fitting bra, especially when doing vigorous exercises. Almost half of all women wear the wrong brassière size so do get your size checked and then stick to it. Only wear 'fun' bras for short periods — they don't have the support of an everyday bra. By doing these things you'll put less stretch on the internal supportive structures of the breast and should keep a youthful, good-looking bust longer. Remember though that bras can never actually improve the breast — they can only delay the inevitable happening for a while.

2. Do frequent (preferably daily) exercises to strengthen the muscles under the bust. Two good ones are mentioned on page 201 and here is another. Sit straight with your stomach in and feet flat on the floor. Hold two large books at arm's length and bring them back to your chest. Straighten your arms and hold the books out there for a moment or two. Repeat the procedure as many times as you can for a minute or so.

3. Quite frankly, apart from ensuring that any unsightly hairs around the nipples are removed regularly, the breasts need very little special care. If you enjoy your partner putting cream on your breasts or massaging them, so well and good but there is no need to do so. The skin of the breasts need no special care compared with that of the rest of the body.

4. Avoid cranky treatments, massages and other miracle cures. Most of them are frankly useless and probably only work at all (if

they ever do) because of the exercises so many of them suggest should be done along with the treatment.

In spite of having devoted a whole chapter of the book to 'some common problems' we don't want to give the impression that a woman's breasts are constantly besieged with medical, aesthetic and cosmetic problems because this simply isn't the case. The vast majority of women do absolutely nothing to their breasts but simply treat them like the rest of their body.

CHAPTER 10

Bras

The history of bras

Although most of today's women see a bra as an everyday part of their wardrobe and wear one almost all the time, the bra is in fact a fairly recent invention in the history of clothes and fashion. The history of underwear and fashion is closely intertwined but fashion in clothes is a peculiarly Western art form and probably only dates from about the Middle Ages onwards.

The word 'bra' is, of course, the shortened form of the word brassière. The Oxford English Dictionary claims that 'brassière' was only introduced in 1912 but it was undoubtedly used before this in the USA. No one knows why the word came into existence because although it is French it is not a word the French use for a piece of woman's underwear. In French a *brassière* is an infant's under-bodice. The French word for a brassière is *soutien-gorge*. Perhaps the Americans first adopted or created the word brassière but whoever did so the popular name for the garment ('bra') was first used in about 1937 and is now commonly used by everyone.

In order to understand about bras we need to look at the history of underwear generally.

Ancient peoples wore loose-fitting skins and clothes and even in the sophisticated world of classical Greece men and women were still wearing clothes of draped and folded lengths of material. Both the ancient Greeks and Egyptians wore two layers of clothing but neither could be said to be real underwear as we know it. Female statues of the time show nothing being worn under these lengths of cloth but writings of the time tell of bands of linen or kid wrapped around the waist or chest to shape and control them. A band called a mastodeton (breast band) was also worn around the bust, probably to flatten it. So the Greeks probably invented the very earliest brassière.

As the centuries passed very little change took place in the design of women's clothes until about 1100 when the loose tunic-style dress began to be drawn tightly to the body with lacing at the sides and the back. For the first time, women's clothes became waisted. No one knows why this change should have suddenly occurred but it has been suggested that the grip of the Church was weakening and that a more secular 'modern' outlook on sex meant that women felt they could reveal their true sexual shape. This movement has continued with various hiccoughs until the present day when tight-fitting jeans which separate and emphasize the buttocks and moulded 'no-bras' bras which do the same for the breasts have made women's outlines more sexually explicit than ever before.

As women's clothes became more shaped in the twelfth century, underwear took on an importance simply because many women were not naturally the shape that the fashions dictated. By the second half of the sixteenth century stiff bodices were being worn and whalebone was used to make rigid corsets which encased the abdomen from hips to bust.

In the late eighteenth century the elegant fashions which included petticoats, corsets, smocks, elaborate headdresses, hats and hairstyles were outmoded within a decade and the vogue was for slim, high-waisted muslin or cotton gowns which clung to the figure and needed a minimum of underwear. It has been suggested that the French Revolution was responsible for this abrupt change in ideas about women's clothing. Class distinctions were being eroded and a classless form of clothing adopted. In fact richer materials – silks, satins and so on – were actually banned for a while at this time. This simple form of dress was reflected by a simple type of underwear and many women of the time did away with corsets altogether.

Regency styles included slim sheaths. With these came the 'bust improvers' – an invention which led *The Times* to say in 1799: 'The fashion for false bosoms has at least this utility, that it compels our fashionable fair to wear something.' These false bosoms were usually called 'bosom friends' or 'waxen bosoms' and they soon disappeared only to return in Victorian times.

The corset reared its head again and was to remain popular until well into this century when women found other ways of supporting stockings and rebelled against constricting artificial shapers. In the early nineteenth century corsets began, for the first time, to have cup-shaped sections built into their tops. Before this they had either pushed the bust up from underneath or been high enough to flatten it. In 1816 the strangely named Divorce Corset was invented. This separated the breasts one from the other using a padded triangle of steel between them. It had little effect though on fashion and the shelf-like Victorian bust continued to be the style women most wanted.

Until the middle of the nineteenth century such changes as had occurred in women's fashions had been made on the grounds of 'more natural' being 'more beautiful'. At about this time the female emancipation movement was getting under way and women were pushing for freedom in many areas of their lives. In 1880 the National Dress Society was established to promote the cause of health, comfort and sense in dress, especially in women's dress. It condemned all the excesses of previous eras such as tight lacing, high heels and all clothes that trussed women up like turkeys. It removed corsets from its list of approved underwear but allowed a firm bodice to support the bust. It also laid down a maximum weight limit for the total weight of all a woman's underwear. At 7 lb (about 3 kg) the average modern woman would feel somewhat overburdened!

The fashionable Edwardian was solemnly dressed on the outside but underneath things were very different. Beautiful underwear was an essential part of the Edwardian lady's wardrobe and led one expert of the day to say, 'Exquisite lingerie forms the foundation of the wardrobe of the woman of refinement', and to go on to advise that one-fifth of one's clothing allowance be put aside for lingerie and corsets.

But even though this was an important trend in underwear it was very much influenced by the restricting and unnatural shapes of current Edwardian fashion. Strangely it was the new-found interest in science and health so prevalent among the Victorians that started the real revolution against any form of restricting garments. Designers started to make corsets that would aid health instead of harming it but even so many women clung to the old styles, often at considerable personal discomfort.

World War I saw women in uniform and doing physical work in military and civilian settings and it was at this time that bras began to catch on in a big way. Women found that the support that a bra gave was not only practical but comfortable and in 1915 it was said that 'a pretty bust bodice or a brassière counts quite as much an essential as a corset'.

After the war women had a different outlook on life. They had worked alongside men and proved themselves to be valuable members of society in a way which they had previously been unable to do. They soon had the vote and the fashion was for women to look more like men. The bosom was flattened and whole body corsets encased women from above the bust down to below the hips. This boyish figure not only eliminated the breasts but also the waist. The brassière of the day became a simple breast flattener. At this time many famous corset manufacturers started to make bras and by the mid 1920s, busts and waistlines were again coming into fashion.

The first mass-produced shaping and separating bra was born around the mid 1920s and deep bust cups were developed in 1928. This heralded a completely new concept in brassière design. They ceased to be artificial 'bust makers' or 'bust flatteners' and started to control what women's breasts were naturally like. Along with this went the realization by corsetry manufacturers that they had, for the first time ever, to give some thought to the different shapes of different women. Up until this time women were expected to squeeze into what was available.

It was the corsetry company Berlei, at that time operating in Australia, which first measured women's figures scientifically. They took five thousand women and made twenty-six measurements on each. Their results, analysed and published in 1928, showed that women fell into five figure types regardless of their build. Berlei repeated this research in 1976. Such knowledge led the company to bring in sizing of underwear when they started up in the UK in 1930 and soon the skilled corsetry fitter became a part of the fashion scene. In 1935 the USA company Warner Bros introduced cup fittings A, B, C and D as today, but their system of sizing wasn't generally adopted for some years. Up until 1940 in Britain bust sizes alone were being used although in 1939 bust cup sizes were recorded as 'junior', 'medium', 'full' and 'full with wide waist'.

The strapless bra came in 1938 but didn't become really popular until the 1950s. The wired bra too came in just before the war. Padded bras had already been in use for a decade. In 1939 bras were already beginning to suggest the high bosom look of the post-war years and very pointed, conical breasts were all the rage in the 1950s when screen idols such as Jane Russell were the sex goddesses of the day. This obsession with artificially shaped and pointed breasts almost certainly originated in the USA and even today there is evidence that the US male is still much more interested in breasts as erotic zones than are his other Western brothers.

The 1950s fashion for prominent, pointed, conical breasts produced an enormous demand for false breasts of all kinds. For those whom Nature had 'let down' there were 'falsies' of many different designs. In 1955 it was estimated that one-quarter of all women were wearing 'cuties' or 'falsies' and all kinds of bust makers were very popular. There were even inflatable ones that could be blown up to the desired size! Unfortunately, they tended to deflate during air travel.

As women became more liberated in the 1960s, this pandering to men's extraordinary ideas of the 'ideal' bust became a thing of the past. Fashion being what it is, though, the erotic focus simply shifted elsewhere – this time to the legs. The 1960s saw mini skirts become popular, especially among young women. This fashion exposed women's legs up to the middle of the thigh and on mounting stairs or indeed doing almost anything active, their thighs and even more were on public view. Clearly stockings revealing a gap of flesh couldn't be worn without looking ugly, and tights (panti-hose) literally and metaphorically filled the gap. Knickers had to be brief to look nice under a mini skirt and the well-dressed woman of the 1960s wore only a bra, pants and tights under her outer clothes. This move to less and less underwear, both in number of pieces and in weight, has now spread to women of all ages.

In the mid 1960s, fashions such as the 'see-through' look and the no-bra bra were gimmicks but laid an important base for the development of the bra and indeed underwear generally. The idea was growing fast that women wanted some sort of underwear but that it had to be light, easy to wear and to look after and as nearly invisible as possible. Panti-girdles and corselettes became unpopular especially among the young and corset manufacturers were forced to produce much prettier, yet still supporting garments. They were greatly helped in this by the discovery of techniques that allowed man-made fibres to be moulded. This means that a woman can wear a pretty, lightweight garment that still has the strength to control her bust. This, for the moment anyway, is what fashion dictates as being desirable. We fully expect that a woman reading this book in 1999 will have as good a laugh at us as we have had at our ancestors' expense.

Bras Today

Today the bra market is very big business indeed with nearly £150 million worth being bought in the UK alone each year. British women in 1979 bought 45 million bras and there is an increasing market for luxury and 'fun' bras.

We have seen already that fashions in outer and underwear have changed considerably as the role of women in society has changed and women's demands from their bras reflect this today. More than a half of all married women work in the UK today and most women say that they like a comfortable, controlling bra to wear for daytime and for working in.

Contrary to popular belief and, indeed, male fantasy, the vast majority of women of all ages still prefer to wear a bra most of the time. Even among those who responded to our survey (and we saw on page 21 that these were atypical in certain ways), only 21 per cent said they did not usually wear a bra. Sixteen per cent of women, however, said they went without a bra all the time and 62 per cent 'sometimes'. Most women who go bra-less do so only in the evenings and on social occasions.

There is no doubt that the main reasons women wear bras today are for comfort and support and this was borne out in our survey. Experienced bra fitters and salespeople say that the thing women dislike most of all about their breasts is if they bounce when they move or run. Undoubtedly the reasons behind this are both comfort and looks and today's woman buys a bra for these two reasons first and foremost.

A great deal of research has been done on women's attitudes to bras and their requirements of them. This shows that women are, almost without exception, very bust conscious. They regard their bust as a manifest sign of their sex, sexuality and role definition. Almost all women know what 'shape' they want to be and the 'look' they want to obtain from a bra. It's often difficult for a woman to describe very coherently what this look is, involving as it does the appearance of the bust as she looks at herself in the mirror (front-on and in profile) and from above. Every woman has her own idea of how she looks best and this develops as a result of her psychosexual rearing and her concept of her body image. Some women are so displeased with their breasts that they can see no hope in the purchase of a pretty bra and others buy bras by the dozen because they enjoy their breasts and see them as important both to themselves and their partners.

Women dress first for their own comfort and next to be attractive to men. Most women say that they want to 'make the most of what they've got' but there are limits to what they'll do to achieve this. Women by and large don't want too much uplift, exposure or cleavage which are seen as tarty, coarse and whorish; don't want to use too much in the way of artificial aids to get the look they want; and don't like 'no-bra' looks which leave nothing to the imagination.

Most women remember very vividly the first bra they bought and this is usually closely bound up with their memories of their early adolescence and emerging sexuality. Breast development is re-membered by many women as a time of teasing by their peer group and even by their father and many women have unfavourable memories of their first bra because it was disliked, unsuitable, too functional, chosen by mother or sister, or even a 'hand-me-down'. There is no ideal age to start wearing a bra, though the first one is usually worn between the ages of eleven and thirteen. A young girl should wear a bra when she feels she's ready for one. There really is no other yardstick. If her friends wear bras, and she wants to as well even if she doesn't actually need one, let her have one: it won't do any harm, which is more than can be said about fighting over the subject.

Research shows that young teenagers want the following from a bra. First, it must be comfortable with no restrictions so that the girl is as unaware as possible that she is wearing it. This is interesting in view of the psychosexual development of girls at this age because they have an ambivalence towards their growing breasts, as we saw on page 94. Most young girls want to wear a bra but they don't want to be physically or psychologically aware of it. The second thing that these young girls want from a bra is prettiness and a fun-like character. If only more mothers reaslized this many girls' memories of their first bra would be a lot happier. Young girls want a soft, rounded shape and certainly do not want a bra to flatten them in any way. Good separation was one of the main points mentioned by 12-13-year-olds in one survey and though they didn't want a cleavage they didn't want a bra that squeezed their breasts together either.

By the age of fourteen most girls are less embarrassed about their breasts and are beginning to see them as part of their sexual display.

At this age girls begin to want a bra that emphasizes what they have and bras that create a cleavage are in demand.

By and large, adult women want two sorts of bra: a 'sensible' type to be worn every day and a more attractive one to be worn in the evenings. The fun type is usually less supportive, in lighter colours, produces more of a cleavage, covers less of the breast and may be frankly erotic. Today's woman has on average six to eight bras in regular use and several others for special occasions.

Research has shown that women want bras which are:
* Machine-washable (see below under 'Caring for bras').
* Made of synthetic fabric such as Lycra, which is flexible, light-weight, easily washed and durable. Cotton bras are popular for sporting and hot weather use but are generally seen as old-fashioned and lacking the properties of Lycra.
* So constructed as to have elastic or stretch straps that are wide enough not to cut into the shoulders.
* Fitted with adjustable straps.
* Designed with low-cut sides to eliminate discolouring due to underarm perspiration.
* Without rough seams which can cause pain on the sensitive skin of the pre-menstrual breast.
* Easy to fasten. Most women with back-fastening bras fasten them at the front and move the bra round to its correct position. Most women prefer back-fastening bras, maintaining that the front fastener always shows through clothes and they are worried that the fastner will pop open.
* Made with no rigid reinforcement. When support is required most women would rather have an underband and preferably one with sufficient width not to dig into the body yet not so wide as to roll back on itself.
* Not evident through outerwear. In other words, one which looks natural.

The biggest selling bra in the world is the Gossard Wonderbra which is slightly padded, very pretty, gives some degree of uplift and good separation.

Things which annoy women about bras are:
* A lack of sizing continuity from brand to brand and even within some brands.
* A lack of mid-cup sizes (such as AB or BC).

* The fact that just as they get to 'know' a good bra it is taken off the market.
* Too few colours.
* A lack of variety of designs, colours and styles for the over-36-inch bust.
* The impossibility of finding a pretty bra in the larger cup sizes.
* The lack of knowledge of sales staff in many shops.

Buying a bra

Women buy several bras a year, mostly from self-service outlets. This gives the woman the advantage of being able to choose what she wants without any 'interference' from a corsetry fitter but also has its drawbacks. The main problem of this method of selling is that it encourages women to buy on impulse and then to be disappointed when they try the bra on at home. Many women have a drawer full of bras they either never or rarely wear simply because they never really fitted in the first place. Human nature being what it is, most women don't bother to take these bras back to the shop and so end up wasting their money.

Big stores and specialist shops have trained corsetry fitters but most young women and many older ones don't like the idea of someone advising them on bra buying and so fail to get the benefit of their advice. Corsetry fitters do know how to find the best bra for you and it's probably well worth while being measured professionally every few years even if most of the time you buy bras 'off the peg'. The main advantage of seeking the help of a fitter is that she will know her stock and will save you a lot of wasted time and possibly even return journeys to the shop to take back bras you're not happy with. She will know if a particular maker's B cup is on the large (or small) side and will be especially valuable if you are anything other than a standard size.

A large number of women buy bras by mail order from a catalogue. This can work very well if you measure yourself carefully as instructed in the catalogue. The main advantage is that once the bra comes you can try it on in the comfort of your home, try it under various clothes you intend wearing with it and see what your partner thinks of it. If you don't like it you can send it back and have your money refunded.

In the UK one store group, Marks and Spencer, sells over a third of all the bras sold nationally – the remainder are sold in departmental stores, high street markets, by mail order and in specialist shops. Most women buy more than one bra at a time and try when possible to match the basic colour to tone with that of the garment it is to go under. It appears that the pleasure of finding a well-fitting, attractive bra encourages a woman who only went out to buy one garment to buy more. This is especially true of colours within one style.

When it comes to buying a bra women still choose white most often. Skin-coloured and cream are the next most popular colours. Why women continue to buy white bras when they know that they discolour on repeated laundering and with the use of deodorants isn't known but it may well be because of the 'white is purity' concept of their upbringing. Although cotton keeps its colour better than do synthetic fibres women don't like cotton bras. It appears that if there is a matching pair of pants to go with the bra most women will buy both.

Wired bras are very popular but some women and indeed corsetry fitters worry about the dangers of wearing them especially if they are wrongly sized. When buying a wired bra be sure that it is very comfortable and that no wire digs into the breast at any part of the bra. Although folklore has it that wired bras can cause cancer, this is not so. They can produce a localized thickening of connective and fibrous tissue if they rub over one place repeatedly but this is not at all like a cancer and will often disappear if the bra is discarded.

Natural shapes are currently all the vogue yet most women say that they want a bra which enhances what they have. Young girls and teenagers are averse to any bra that shows the nipple through either the bra itself or through outer clothes and older women have mixed feelings about this. Many like a sheer bra that shows the nipple colour and contour through but don't want this to show through their clothes. Very few women it seems like their nipples to show (especially when their breasts are cold) through clothes.

By and large, elasticated straps are preferable to other types mainly because they are more comfortable to wear and don't slip. On the negative side, elasticated straps are often the first part of a bra to discolour and wear out.

Unless you are buying a brand and size of bra with which you are totally familiar you should always try it on in the shop. Here's what to do, assuming you know your size.

* Select the style and colour you like.
* Take it to a dressing-room and take all the clothes off your top half. You can't try on a bra over a sweater or anything else.
* Put the bra on in the way you always do, fixing to the outermost eye. If it fits well like this when new you can always tighten it one eye as the bra stretches on repeated laundering.
* See that it fits snugly around your body and lies flat. It should not stand away from the body between the breasts.
* See that the bust is fully contained within each cup. Any wrinkling at the point or gaping at the side of the cup means that the cup is too *small*. If there is 'all over wrinkling' the cup is too large. With either of these wrinkling problems try another *cup* but keep the same *bra* size.
* See that flesh doesn't bulge over the top of the cups (there's nothing worse than the 'four breast' look), under your arms or across your back. If flesh bulges underneath the underbust band perhaps a long line bra would be better.
* If the bra is underwired see that the wiring lies flat on the chest wall and doesn't dig in anywhere.
* Check that the straps are wide enough for comfort. Are they adjusted to the right height?
* Check that the bottom of the bra goes around the chest horizontally and is not pulled up at the back. Adjust the straps as necessary to achieve this.
* Lastly, sit down in the bra. A well-fitting bra should feel good when standing or sitting. When you are seated the underband (if there is one) shouldn't roll up; you shouldn't spill out of the top of the bra; and no wires should dig in anywhere.

The corsetry trade suggests that when you are standing the centre of the nipple should be on a level with the middle of your upper arm. No matter what type of breast you have, if you end up in a bra that does this you'll look good in it under clothes. When we say 'look good' we mean, of course, society's currently held view on what constitutes 'good' in this context – and this is purely arbitrary, changing as it does with vogues and fashion.

All of this assumes you know what size you are. But supposing you don't, how do you measure yourself for a bra? It's really quite simple.

* Take a centimetre measuring tape (bras are now all in Eurosizes

even though most women still think in inches). Take your top and bra off and stand in front of a mirror.

* To get the chest size (the '34' part of the old 34B bra size) take the tape around your chest so that it is completely horizontal and lies *under* your breasts. This can be tricky to do on your own because your bust may need lifting out of the way and it's not always easy to see if the tape is horizontal. This is why it's best to be measured by a fitter while you gently lift your bust.

This table shows you what English size bra you'll need for each metric (Eurosize) measurement.

Table of metric bra sizing and English equivalents.

Underbust measurement (cm)	Appropriate bra size	English size (inches)
68/72	70	32
73/77	75	34
78/82	80	36
83/87	85	38
88/92	90	40
93/97	95	42
98/102	100	44

x When measuring, don't pull the tape too tight but just tight enough to simulate the normal tightness of the bra. You now know your chest size and this should not change much from make to make of bra. Once you have the chest size in centimetres (say 80), look across the table to find your Eurosize bra (80) and then across one more column to find the English equivalent (36 inches). The measurement under your breast in centimetres converted to inches is not the same thing at all. In other words, if you measure yourself under the bust and you are 33 inches, for example, this does *not* mean you'll need a bra with an English size of 33. Stick to measuring in centimetres and do the conversion using the table and you can't go wrong.

Having obtained an underbust measurement in centimetres this is only useful for bra measurements. Whenever you measure yourself for a blouse, clothes, slips and so on always take the *overbust* (measured in a good bra) size. The underbust measurement has been found to be most accurate for bra measurements but not for outer clothes.

* Now to cup size. Assessing cup sizes is very difficult even for an experienced fitter and no ready-made formulae are of any use at all. Experienced fitters say that women always overestimate their cup size just as they always underestimate their hip size! If your breasts are very small and have absolutely no droop then an A cup will probably be right for you. If you have very large pendulous breasts you'll probably need a D cup and if you're in between you'll need a B or a C. Most women wear B or C cups and you'll have to see which is best for you with any one brand by trial and error. The assistants won't mind you taking a B and a C bra in any style you try.

All of this procedure can be done in a few minutes by a trained fitter. Although many women don't like the idea of 'being poked about' or even showing their bodies to other women it is probably well worth while. There are thousands of fitters all over the country and all specialist shops and many big stores have them. They are by no means always grey-haired matrons any more and are trained never to touch your breasts during their measuring and fitting. They will help you with any request but are especially useful if you are overweight, have a very large bust, have had a mastectomy, are pregnant or nursing, have breasts of unequal size or want a specialist bra. Many specialist bras do not conform to normal sizings and can be difficult to fit on your own. Just because you go to a fitter don't feel bound to buy anything unless you like it. Most stores and specialist shops use their fitters as an advisory service to their customers and not simply for selling the latest bra.

It probably makes sense not to buy a bra in the four or five days before a period because most women's breasts swell at this time and they end up buying a bra in too large a cup size for the other twenty-five days of the month. Some women like to keep a few bras with larger cup sizes for these few days of the month when their breasts swell. While on the subject of breast swelling remember that during pregnancy your breasts will swell and that by about the fourth or fifth month you'll probably be out of your ordinary bras and into larger sizes. Most women find they need a bra one cup size and one bra size bigger. So if you were a 34B before you were pregnant you'll probably need a 36C. When trying on a maternity bra always get one that is comfortable when it is done up on the tightest eye so as to leave room for expansion. Whilst on the subject of increasing bust size it's interesting to note that over the last five years women's average bust size has increased. Five years ago the most popular bra size was 34B, now it's 36C. No one knows for sure why this should be but increased food intake, the Pill and more physical exercise are possible factors. This is proving advantageous to the woman with a larger bust because there are now more pretty bras that will fit her.

Caring for your bra

Modern bra fabrics last well and keep looking good for months or years. However, if you want to keep your bra looking and feeling good, here are some general rules.

* Never wear a bra for more than a day or two so that it doesn't get too soiled.
* Always hand wash with soap.
* Never force dry but let the bra dry naturally. Force drying damages the elastic parts and discolours the bra itself.
* Check on your bras every now and then to look for signs of wear. If a wire begins to push through, mend it if possible. If the bra feels at all uncomfortable get rid of it and replace it.

Why wear a bra at all?

As we have already said, the vast majority of women wear a bra most of the time and they do so for comfort and support. Some women resent the thought that a male-dominated society expects them to wear a bra so that their breasts conform to some notional 'ideal' (set by men) and so do not wear one at all. Interestingly, a fair proportion of women over fifty-five don't wear bras but their motives for not doing so are probably very different.

One of the commonest questions we are asked is: 'Is it dangerous to go bra-less?' The answer is, of course, 'No'. It may be uncomfortable if you have large breasts but no physical damage results from going bra-less. Similarly, there's no harm in wearing a well-fitting bra either. Going without a bra for years will mean that your breasts will droop but this is no tragedy. After all, a woman's breasts tend to droop as she ages anyway so all a good bra can do is to help delay the process a little.

If you have a mole that is rubbed or scratched by the straps, the underbust band or any other part of your bra it is worth having it removed because on repeated irritation such moles can, though rarely, become malignant.

Some women are allergic to the elastic materials from which certain straps are made but this can be easily overcome by changing brands.

If you have large breasts or if you are pregnant you may find it more comfortable to wear a bra at night. Some women with breast pain (see page 105) also find that wearing a bra for twenty-four hours a day is more comfortable.

However well-fitting your bra is, it will never actually improve your bust in the long term. As soon as you remove a bra any good it does is lost. Having said this, though, one could say that a bra does permanent good if it prevents stretch marks and droop or delays them for many years. Very large breasts, the pregnant and lactating breast, the painful breast and the breast immediately after cosmetic surgery really are helped by wearing a snug-fitting bra.

Lactating (breastfeeding) women sometimes find special nursing bras useful, especially those that undo in front to enable one breast at a time to be given to the baby. Other women, however, manage perfectly well with an ordinary bra and pull the cups up or down over the breast to feed. Just because you are breastfeeding doesn't necessarily mean you'll have to buy nursing bras.

Women who have had a mastectomy can buy special bras with a pocket on the affected side into which a prosthesis can be placed (see page 191). This means that when wearing a bra many mastectomy patients look perfectly normal when otherwise naked and certainly do so when dressed.

So whether or not you wear a bra and what bra you wear is entirely up to you. There is no medical argument either for or against wearing one and thankfully we live in a sensible society (on these matters anyway) that doesn't much care one way or the other. Men like to see women — in well-fitting bras or without them — and research shows that other women don't mind either way. The fact is that as a species we do have rather larger breasts for our body size than most animals and most women feel more comfortable in a bra. Countless millions of women around the world don't wear bras at all, though, so clearly bras are cultural garments and nothing more.

CHAPTER 11

The male breast

At birth the male breast is exactly like that of the female and can, as we shall see, also produce milk for a few days. In fact the breasts of both sexes stay much the same until puberty when the female breast develops and the male one does not. Just why males should have breasts at all is a mystery of nature but males certainly do have breast tissue which is mainly made up of ducts and blood vessels and not milk-producing cells. Having said this, though, the adult male breast *can* produce milk and men have been recorded as feeding babies (albeit extremely rarely) throughout history. To all intents and purposes, however, the male breast has no known function and isn't subject to cyclical influences as is the female breast. Certain changes do, though, occur in the male breast. The only phenomena worth consideration in a book such as this are sexual arousal, deformities present from birth, nipple discharge, swellings and cancer.

The male breast as a sex organ

There has been very little research on this subject but it is widely reported by men during psychosexual interviews that breasts do play a sexual role in some of them. Most men enjoy the sensation produced by a woman's body pressing against their chest but this is probably no different from the pleasure they'd get if she did the same to another part of their body.

A man's nipples are often pleasantly sensitive to the touch and it is well known that many men's nipples erect when stimulated sexually just as women's do. This is not too surprising since micro-dissection of the male breast reveals exactly similar nerve endings as in the female breast. Some men manipulate their nipples when they masturbate, just as some women do. Having said this, though, most men are surprisingly indifferent to their nipples as centres of sexual pleasure. To be fair to those men who do enjoy nipple sensations it should be pointed out that most of us are not good at touching and arousing each other using touch. Many women complain that their men don't do what they most enjoy when it comes to breast stimulation in love-making yet we all perceive the female breast as a pleasure-centre for both men and women. We suspect that more men would enjoy their nipples being stimulated but unless they tell their partners what they'd like, how can they expect them to know? Enough men say how sexually pleasant (if not actively arousing) it is to have a woman stimulate their nipples to make it worth while bringing the subject up within a loving relationship. It's much like everything else in sexuality: unless you've tried it you can't know if you're going to enjoy it.

Birth deformities

Those that occur in the female breast (see page 123) can also occur in the male. In fact, extra nipples are found more commonly in men than in women. When they do occur though they have no underlying breast tissue as sometimes occurs in women. This means that no treatment is necessary at puberty because no development occurs, as it does in girls. Extra nipples may be removed for purely cosmetic reasons but many men never seek treatment for this minor abnormality.

There can be a complete absence of one breast in men just as in women but this rarely causes any problems because quite obviously the loss is not as noticeable as it is in women.

Nipple discharge

Although the male breast is an organ with no apparent function it can produce a discharge from the nipple and this can be very worrying to men. Milk secretion sometimes occurs in a newborn baby boy for the first few days after birth. This 'witch's milk', as it has been called, is produced as a result of the effect of the mother's hormones on the baby boy's breast tissue. A milk duct can become blocked leading to an accumulation of this milk in the breast which can then become infected. Such a breast abscess in a newborn baby boy is, however, very rare.

The nipple of a pubertal boy can also discharge fluid but this is most often a part of a condition known as gynaecomastia (see below).

Any nipple discharge in a boy should be reported to a doctor at once because it could be a sign of breast cancer (see below).

Breast swelling (gynaecomastia − 'female breast')

Gynaecomastia, breast swelling in a male, is common and has many causes. It can be a normal physiological phenomenon or a sign of underlying disease. The swelling can be very marked or barely visible and on occasions can be so severe as to produce a breast which looks just like a woman's. If you're thinking that this must be a very rare condition indeed just bear in mind that about three-quarters of all pubertal boys have some degree of breast swelling − often to their extreme embarrassment.

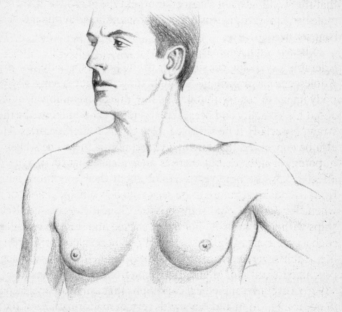

Gynaecomastia.

There are many causes of gynaecomastia. The enlarged breasts of a baby are caused by his mother's high hormone levels. Young boys on the other hand almost never have breast swelling but swelling around the time of puberty is extremely common, as we have seen, and indeed could be thought of as normal.

Pubertal gynaecomastia usually comes on between the ages of twelve and seventeen and takes the form of a discrete, rubbery, often tender disc of tissue underneath the nipples. The young lad is often unaware of the condition unless it is gross. The swelling can be one-sided or affect both sides. Only about a quarter of affected boys have bilateral swelling. When one side only is affected it is usually the left. Very rarely the nipple and areola enlarge but the formation of a truly female-looking breast is uncommon.

No one knows what causes this self-limiting condition but it usually disappears within two years at the most. Only boys who have swellings for longer than this may need surgical treatment. Hormones have been blamed for such swellings but there is no conclusive evidence on this as yet. Many boys and, indeed, their parents need reassurance that the swelling is not a cancer or other type of growth. Cancer of the male breast is rare anyway and is almost unknown at this age. A biopsy is never needed.

Pubertal gynaecomastia, quite understandably, causes considerable psychological suffering to the boy, especially if it is gross. Adolescence is a difficult enough time without having a distorted body image to cope with too. The boy already has ambivalent feelings about his sexuality and breast enlargement can sometimes be the final straw, especially if he is teased a lot by his contemporaries. He may also be concerned that having gynaecomastia means he's likely to be impotent or infertile but there is no evidence that this is true. Many affected boys become very anxious about their condition, withdraw from friendships, refuse to be seen naked at school, get out of sports whenever possible, and some become clinically depressed. Relationships with girls are halted or never started and some experts feel that such a poor start can affect a person psychosexually for the rest of his life. Such severely affected boys need the help of a psychologist or psychiatrist and a lot of understanding from their families.

There are several medical conditions that can cause gynaecomastia in adult men. Men and boys with certain malformations of the penis and testis suffer more frequently from the condition than would be expected. Undescended testes and hypospadias are the two commonest examples of such conditions. Gynaecomastia is also a part of the Klinefelter syndrome. These men have small testes, produce no sperms and have a special XXY type of chromosome formation in their cells. Such men also have a higher than normal chance of developing cancer of the breast.

Other diseases associated with gynaecomastia include testicular tumours, tumours of the adrenal gland, cirrhosis of the liver, severe starvation, lung cancer, tuberculosis and overactivity of the thyroid gland. Breast enlargement is also often seen in paraplegics.

Drugs are a common cause of male breast enlargement and both male and female hormone therapy can cause it. It is most often seen after the use of female sex hormones to treat cancer of the prostate gland. Breast enlargement in these patients can be prevented with small doses of radiation to the breasts. As well as these sex hormone drugs, spironolactone, reserpine, phenothiazines, methyldopa, meprobamate, diethylpropion, amphetamines, ergotamine, diphenylhydantoin and marijuana can all cause breast enlargement as can digitalis and isoniazid. Withdrawal of the drug produces a normal breast within a few weeks.

Old men can get a kind of senile gynaecomastia. This usually takes the form of a small tender lump under the areola. It usually disappears spontaneously within a few months. In many ways it is rather like pubertal gynaecomastia and causes considerable anxiety. At this age though the fear is that it might be a cancer.

Gynaecomastia can produce three symptoms: a lump, a discharge from the nipple, or pain. Most men complain only of a lump and nipple discharge is rare.

Before we look at the treatments that are available let's just look at pseudo-gynaecomastia. Many men are obese today and the breast in men (as in women) is a common place for fat to be deposited. Such men have no enlargement of their breast tissue and can be treated by weight reduction alone. However, fatty, pendulous breasts can be so uncomfortable and embarrassing that they may need surgery.

Treatment depends very much upon the cause of the condition. Obviously, breast swelling in the newborn needs no treatment and the vast majority of pubertal boys are normal again within a few months. Breast enlargement in adults though does need to be taken seriously and most men with the condition over the age of twenty-five have something serious going on that is causing the condition. Some of the causes can be treated: for example, a drug can be stopped and another substituted.

Sorting out the causes of adult breast enlargement is a skilful business and must be done by a specialist who knows what he's dealing with. But often there comes a stage when no underlying treatable illness or other cause can be found and the man wants to be freed from his embarrassing deformity. Surgery is the only answer at this stage – no drug treatment does any good at all.

A surgeon can remove the breast tissue and the spare skin on the chest wall and can even reduce the size of the areola if this has overgrown too. The scars are very fine and after a year or so there is almost no evidence of the operation at all. The operation is called a subcutaneous mastectomy and leaves the nipple intact. In this procedure, the enlarged breast tissue is removed from inside the breast and the man's chest returned to normal. It in no way compares with the classical mastectomy performed for female breast cancer. It is not a major procedure and after two to three days in hospital most men are home and on the road to recovery.

Breast cancer

This cancer accounts for only one in a hundred of all breast cancers. In other words, 99 per cent of all breast cancers are in women. However, with over 100,000 new breast cancers a year being found in the USA, for example, this means that more than 1,000 men a year are diagnosed as having this condition – so it's worth knowing about. In Africa male breast cancer is much more common though it's not known why.

The causes of breast cancer in men are as obscure as they are in women. Breast cancer is known to be more common among women whose close female relatives have had cancer of the breast and similar findings are evident in men too, but here the link is between other men with breast cancer in the family. There is no agreement as to whether gynaecomastia is a causative factor in male breast cancer but some surveys suggest that there is a link.

Klinefelter syndrome (see page 237) is definitely associated with a greatly increased incidence of breast cancer and men suffering from this condition are said to have as much breast cancer as do women.

The man who develops breast cancer is on average sixty years old (six to eleven years older than his female counterpart). More cancers are of the left breast than the right and nine out of ten men first complain of a lump. Complaints relating to the nipple and areola are much more common than they are among women, mainly because there is so little mass to the male breast that any cancer affecting it soon affects the nipple and the skin of the breast.

Nipple discharge is a relatively common occurrence, present in one in seven men with breast cancer. The discharge is usually pale, straw-coloured, or tinged with blood. Any such discharge must receive medical attention at once as it indicates an underlying cancer in 75 per cent of men – three times more often than it does in women.

Men seem to put off going to their doctors with a breast lump longer than do women. One major study found that the diagnosis in men was significantly delayed in three-quarters of men and only (!) in two-thirds of women. Anyway, the vast majority of men with breast cancer do not discover their own lump. (Most breast cancers in women, by comparison, are discovered by the woman herself.)

Diagnosing the lump is usually very easy for a doctor though mammography is used when necessary.

Treatment, however, is a confused subject, even by female breast cancer standards. This is partly because it is a rare disease and because many of the surveys that have been done are not comparable. What tends to happen therefore is that men with breast cancer get treated on the basis of what has been learned from experience with women. This may not be ideal.

Radical mastectomy in men is a more difficult procedure than the same operation in women mainly because there is so little tissue there. Just as in female cancer, chemotherapy and/or radiation are used alone or in combination with surgery.

The outlook for any one individual with breast cancer is always difficult to predict but in men the process is even more tricky. Men overall have a poorer outlook than women with breast cancer because the tumour more quickly affects tissues outside the breast. In 1927 the five-year survival rate for men with breast cancer was 19 per cent but today the figure is at least double this. However much of an improvement this may appear, the outlook is still much worse than for women. Young men, it seems, have a worse outlook than older men with the condition.

If, in spite of the initial treatment, the cancer recurs, certain other measures can be used. Just as the ovaries of women with breast cancer can be removed with good effect on the cancer, so also can men's testes be removed to eliminate the effect of male hormones on the tumour. Various other hormone treatments have also been tried but the results are inconclusive. One of the newer tests that is used to decide whether to use drugs or hormones is one that measures the level of specific cell components known as oestrogen receptors. These are tumour cell structures that seem to have an affinity for oestrogens. A positive test means that the tumour is oestrogen-dependent and so might respond to hormone (or anti-hormone) drugs. Such a test can also be used in women with breast cancer. (see page 197).

There seems little doubt that the poor outlook for men with breast cancer could be improved if they went to their doctors as soon as they found a lump or a discharge. Doctors too should be more aware of the condition and should examine the breasts of all men over sixty when the opportunity arises.

Index

ALSO BY DR ANDREW STANWAY
IN GRANADA PAPERBACKS

WHY US?

a commonsense guide for the childless

Why Us? is a cry from the heart ... an emotional plea from all
those people who long to share in nature's simplest gift of all,
parenthood.

Infertility has too long been kept in the shadows. Here Dr
Andrew Stanway takes a fresh, honest look at the subject, and
finds that simple, self-help measures can commonly work
wonders. And when infertility persists, Dr Stanway is a caring
guide to the many forms of treatment available. Where
conventional medical opinion is so often distant, *Why Us?* gives
reassurance and invaluable practical advice, and casts an
objective eye over future prospects for the childless couple in
this age of test-tube babies.

£1.95

A DICTIONARY OF OPERATIONS:
A Handbook for Patients

Most people going into hospital for an operation feel that they
do not know enough about what is going to happen to them,
either in the theatre or on the ward. Now Dr Andrew Stanway
has produced a lucid and commonsense book that answers the
kind of questions that people find it hard to ask, or to get
answered in a way that they can understand.

Part 1
Includes chapters on

WAITING TO GO INTO HOSPITAL
WHO'S WHO IN THE HOSPITAL
BEFORE THE OPERATION
AFTER THE OPERATION
YOUR LEGAL RIGHTS AND HOW TO COMPLAIN
PRIVATE SURGERY
CHILDREN IN HOSPITAL
WHAT TO TAKE IN
WHAT IT IS LIKE BEING A SURGICAL PATIENT
IN THE OPERATING THEATRE
VISITORS
GOING HOME AND CONVALESCING
NATIONAL HEALTH SERVICE BENEFITS

Part 2
CONSISTS OF AN A–Z OF OPERATIONS

Part 3
GIVES AN ALPHABETICAL LIST OF PROCEDURES
AND INVESTIGATIONS

In short, *A Dictionary of Operations* is all you need to know to
make a stay in hospital, be it your own or that of a friend or
relative, more understandable and less stressful.

£2.50

A SELECTION OF SEXOLOGY BOOKS FROM GRANADA PAPERBACKS

GF3981

HEALTH AND FITNESS BOOKS NOW AVAILABLE IN
GRANADA PAPERBACKS

W H Bates
Better Eyesight Without Glasses — £1.95 ☐

Christine Beels
The Childbirth Book — £1.95 ☐

Desmonde Dunne
Yoga Made Easy — £1.50 ☐

Laurence E Morehouse & Leonard Gross
Total Fitness — £1.25 ☐
Maximum Performance — 95p ☐

Constance Mellor
Guide to Natural Health — 80p ☐
Natural Remedies for Common ailments — £1.95 ☐

Sonya Richmond
Yoga and Your Health — 95p ☐

Phyllis Speight
Homoeopathy — £1.50 ☐

All these books are available at your local bookshop or newsagent, or can be ordered direct from the publisher. Just tick the titles you want and fill in the form below.

Name _____

Address _____

_____

Write to Granada Cash Sales
PO Box 11, Falmouth, Cornwall TR10 9EN.

Please enclose remittance to the value of the cover price plus:

UK 45p for the first book, 20p for the second book plus 14p per copy for each additional book ordered to a maximum charge of £1.63.

BFPO and Eire 45p for the first book, 20p for the second book plus 14p per copy for the next 7 books, thereafter 8p per book.

Overseas 75p for the first book and 21p for each additional book.

Granada Publishing reserve the right to show new retail prices on covers, which may differ from those previously advertised in the text or elsewhere.

HB881